"Parents of kids with chronic pain, as much or more than other patient populations, want to know what concretely they can do to help their kids. With its focus on psychological techniques, teaching vignettes, and workbook strategies, this book is a unique resource."
—Gerard A. Banez, Ph.D., Cleveland Clinic

"What a truly wonderful book and a gift to families dealing with chronic pain and to the clinicians who care for them! Dr. Coakley's extensive knowledge base, deep clinical experience, and personal warmth and compassion are evident on every page."
—Neil L. Schechter, M.D., Director, Chronic Pain Clinic, Boston Children's Hospital

"Dr. Coakley's book is a superb roadmap and guide for parents of children and adolescents with chronic pain. Her tone and message will resonate with parents from a very broad array of backgrounds and parenting styles. Simply the best book on this subject for parents."
—Charles Berde, M.D., Ph.D., Chief of Pain Medicine, Boston Children's Hospital

"Dr. Coakley has developed a priceless resource that helps parents see the context of the whole child and the important systems—family, school, peers—that play crucial roles in children's experiences of and recovery from chronic pain."
—Deirdre Logan, Ph.D., Harvard Medical School

"After reading this extraordinary and much-needed book by a competent and experienced clinician, parents will feel confident they have the skills, knowledge, and resources necessary to manage their child's chronic pain."
—Grayson N. Holmbeck, Ph. D., Editor of *Journal of Pediatric Psychology*, Loyola University Chicago

When Your Child Hurts

Yale University Press Health & Wellness

A Yale University Press Health & Wellness book is an authoritative, accessible source of information on a health-related topic. It may provide guidance to help you lead a healthy life, examine your treatment options for a specific condition or disease, situate a healthcare issue in the context of your life as a whole, or address questions or concerns that linger after visits to your healthcare provider.

When Your Child Hurts

Effective Strategies to Increase Comfort, Reduce Stress, and Break the Cycle of Chronic Pain

RACHAEL COAKLEY, Ph.D.

Yale UNIVERSITY PRESS

New Haven and London

Published on the foundation established in memory of William Chauncey Williams of the Class of 1822, Yale Medical School, and of William Cook Williams of the Class of 1850, Yale Medical School.

Yale University Press books may be purchased in quantity for educational, business, or promotional use. For information, please e-mail sales.press@yale.edu (U.S. office) or sales@yaleup.co.uk (U.K. office).

Set in Simoncini Garamond type by Newgen North America.
Printed in the United States of America.

ISBN: 978-0-300-20465-0 (paperback; alk. paper)

Library of Congress Control Number 2015941167

A catalogue record for this book is available from the British Library.

This paper meets the requirements of ANSI/NISO Z39.48–1992 (Permanence of Paper).

10 9 8 7 6 5 4 3 2 1

In my office at the Pain Treatment Service at Boston Children's Hospital, my beige, hospital-issued desk is next to the big blue reclining chair where my young patients sit for therapy. One day, I placed on the side of my desk a small white magnet with a simple message from the famous American composer John Cage. It reads, "Begin Anywhere."

This gave several of my patients the idea to post their own inspirational quotations on the side of my desk for everyone to see. Some quotations are from songs, others are from books, and some are just sayings kids have heard along the way. All include words of resilience, strength, and fortitude. For my new patients and their parents, who are frequently struggling the most, the quotations from others who have walked in their shoes are a beacon of hope.

At his very first appointment, Collin, an eight-year-old boy with chronic abdominal pain, carefully studied the side of my desk and then said, "I've got one, too." Many weeks later, when Collin and his family had a new arsenal of strategies for managing his pain, he took a notecard from my desk, grabbed a chunky marker, and wrote: "'It always seems impossible until it's done.' —*Nelson Mandela*."

Contents

Contents

Preface

Mondays are my new clinic day. Each and every Monday I meet two new families for the first time. The stories they tell have different beginnings and middles, but for each the end is the same. "My child has pain and nothing seems to help," parents tell me when I begin my evaluation.

I look at the young person coiled in the big blue recliner chair in my office, and I look at the parents who sit upright on the edges of their seats. For a moment I put myself in their shoes. I recognize that the journey up to this point has often been long and wrought with frustration, heartache, and physical suffering. I understand that families do not come to the multidisciplinary pain clinic where I work without this journey, and I know that hopes are high.

I begin slowly. "Pain is a complicated problem," I say to the parents. I wait until I can catch the eye of the young person who sits in front of me, and I continue. "You are here today because you've already met with many smart doctors, you've already tried medications, you've waited, you've rested, you've done what doctors have told you to do, and you are still hurting." I take a slow deep breath and go on, "Your pain has probably caused a lot of problems in your life. Most people find that pain interferes with school, sleep, friends, activities, concentration, memory, and mood. It also of course causes a lot of worry for you and your parents." I pause. The next thing I have to say is trickier, so I take my time. I have to explain carefully my role within the pain clinic because I am a psychologist, and many people bristle when they are referred to a psychologist for what is obviously a physical problem. "My job here today is to understand how pain has interfered with your life," I say. "I'm not trying to evaluate whether or not your pain is real; I know it's real. I know you're hurting."

I spend a lot of time with my Monday families. I listen to the stories that they tell when they are together as a family, I listen to what the child shares with me when we meet alone, and then I listen to what parents confide when their child is out of the room and they can finally let their guard down. I do a lot of listening on Mondays. I have listened to more than a thousand families tell their stories—stories fraught with frustration, concern, and multiple challenges.

"My pain is horrible and so frustrating; it's ruining my life," states fourteen-year-old Andy, with his eyes firmly fixed on the floor. Andy is a very smart, highly motivated student and an excellent soccer player. He was diagnosed with irritable bowel disease when he was nine, and his family used medication and diet to manage his symptoms for several years. But when Andy turned twelve, he caught a stomach virus and his stomach pain escalated. The stomach virus passed within a few days, but his pain did not resolve. He couldn't eat for over a week and was in severe pain. His gastroenterologist admitted him to the hospital for evaluation and pain control. Unlike the irritable bowel disease flares he experienced in the past, this time his lab work was normal, the endoscopy looked good, and there was no blood in his stool. Andy tried several different medications in the hospital, but none seemed to work. He was discharged from the hospital though he was still in pain. Everyone hoped that his symptoms would resolve within a few weeks. They didn't.

Andy reports that he has had pain almost every day for more than a year and that he was recently diagnosed with functional abdominal pain. He says that his pain interferes with every aspect of his life and that he is doing very poorly in school because he can only attend classes on a limited schedule. He has lost contact with his friends, was cut from the soccer team, and is withdrawn, anxious, and irritable. When Andy steps out of my office, his parents' eyes well up with tears. "He's just not the same kid he used to be; we lost our guy," Andy's Mom shares. I listen carefully. His Mom continues, "You can't imagine how miserable he is; it breaks my heart to see him in so much pain. He cries in pain every night and is exhausted every day. We are all at our wits' end." Tears roll down her cheek and she reaches for a nearby box of tissues.

♦

Kaitlin is ten years old. Her parents describe her as "spunky and spirited." They also note that she's always been very sensitive to pain, so they didn't really believe her when she started complaining of ankle pain four months ago. "It seemed to come out of nowhere," her Mom said. Kaitlin's parents ignored her complaining for three weeks. When the pain persisted, they took her to the pediatrician. She had an x-ray that showed that her ankle bones were intact and later had an MRI that showed no damage to the tissues or tendons. The doctor suggested she wrap her ankle in an ace bandage for support and use crutches for a few weeks to let it rest. But instead of healing, the pain intensified.

Kaitlin now sits in my office with her leg fully extended. She's not wearing a sock or shoe. She's breathing heavily, has fear in her eyes, and reaches out to hold her mother's hand. She's terrified that something, anything, might brush against her foot causing intense pain. She's also terrified that she's going to leave here today without any answers or relief.

"No one understands," she tells me. She and her family have been evaluated by four physicians and have done some research on their own. They know that she has a neuropathic pain condition called complex regional pain syndrome. But this diagnosis has brought more questions than answers. "We know that she needs to do physical therapy to get better, but do you see how much pain she is in? There is no way we can make her do physical therapy in this condition," her Mom states firmly. Her Dad continues, "She does need psychological support because she's falling apart, but talking to her about her pain is not going to help her at this point. She's too far past that." Her Dad sits back in his chair, crosses his arms, and shakes his head in frustration.

◆

Eight-year-old Christopher has struggled with migraine headaches since he was five years old. He also has some sensory-related difficulties and a history of separation anxiety that have presented challenges to his family throughout his early development. Christopher's Mom describes him as a child who has never liked transitions or new situations, has difficulty regulating his behavior especially when he's tired, and is prone to tantrums when he doesn't get his way at home.

Christopher's Mom has a history of migraine headaches, so she is very empathic toward Christopher's pain. As a headache sufferer herself, she understands that stress is often a trigger for his migraine pain, but feels at a loss for how to reduce his stress. His Mom states that she and Christopher's Dad work hard at trying not to upset him so that they can keep his headaches to a minimum. But over the last year his Mom sometimes worries that Christopher is using his headache pain as an excuse to avoid new situations. Even more concerning, she has noticed that his headaches are increasing in frequency despite their best efforts to make his life as stress-free as possible.

◆

Angela's father pushes her rental wheelchair into my office. They are twenty minutes late for their appointment because getting

Angela out of the house today has been a monumental event. Angela is eighteen years old and has widespread body pain that has almost completely disabled her. Her pain started a year ago with some achy joints and a sore back. Given her family history of arthritis, she was whisked through a full rheumatologic evaluation. Testing showed some mild laboratory indicators of inflammation, though she had no clinical evidence of inflammation on exam. She was put on multiple arthritis medications to see if she could experience any relief from her discomfort. She did not. Her pain spread and within a few months she had pain throughout her body. Repeated laboratory assessments showed no signs of arthritis and she was told that her first labs were probably false positives. Angela and her family believe that there is an underlying medical cause for her pain and disability that has yet to be identified. Angela tells me that some doctors have diagnosed her with fibromyalgia and others have told her she has pain amplification syndrome, but she cannot explain these diagnoses in her own words.

Angela's pain has caused major disruptions in her life. She missed the last part of her junior year and her entire senior year at school. Plans for college were put on hold. While gazing at Angela, her Mom says, "Angela is so smart; she was on track to be the valedictorian of her junior year. She's also an accomplished violinist, had the lead role in her school play, and was nominated to be the head of her church youth group." Angela rolls her eyes and mumbles that she hasn't done any of those things in over a year. Angela's mother tries to explain away her daughter's irritable remark, saying that Angela is not herself today because the long car ride aggravated her pain, she didn't sleep well last night, and she had mixed feelings about coming for her evaluation today. Angela's mother admits, "We've been referred to see a psychologist before, but honestly, despite what she's been through, Angela's mood has been pretty positive. Besides, I am always there to support her; I know she would tell me if something was wrong."

I listen carefully to my Monday families because each family needs to be heard. Parents are overwhelmed and exhausted and they hope that within the Pediatric Pain Clinic they will find answers for how to manage their child's persistent pain and disability and will finally be able to move beyond the frustration, confusion, and medical stress they have been experiencing. I understand the sense of helplessness and desperation these families often feel at this particular point in their journey. So it is with great care, after all my listening, that I finally begin to talk to the parents who sit before me.

"I can see that your child is suffering. I know that you are also suffering because, as a parent, I know how deeply you feel your child's pain. I understand that you are frustrated and desperate to help your child through this difficult time. I'm glad you're here."

◆

Current estimates suggest that as many as one of every four children today will experience an episode of pain lasting three months or longer before reaching adulthood. Of those who experience chronic pain, 77 percent will have more than one kind of pain problem. Moreover, the overall incidence of pediatric pain conditions is on the rise; over the past twenty years, reports of chronic headache and abdominal pain syndromes have almost doubled. Whether the increase is attributable to more stress in our children's lives, sedentary lifestyles, genetic pain vulnerabilities, increased attention to pain symptoms, or a combination of factors is currently being debated. But the evidence remains clear: chronic pain is one of the most common problems in pediatrics, with approximately 1.7 million children currently suffering from moderate to severe chronic pain. It also is one of the most expensive pediatric problems, costing 19.5 billion dollars per year—a price tag that places pediatric chronic pain on par with the most expensive pediatric health conditions, namely ADHD and asthma.

If chronic pain is so common and problematic, why do parents often feel so alone in their struggles to learn how to manage it? One reason is that pain is often an invisible problem; most children with chronic pain do not have obvious differences from other children and so the challenges are seldom talked about beyond the child's close family and friends. It is also possible that chronic pain conditions have lacked widespread recognition in pediatrics because historically pediatric pain was viewed through a diagnostic-specific lens. Abdominal pain was researched as part of the field of gastroenterology, headache pain was the domain of neurology, arthritis pain was studied within rheumatology, and so on. An impressive body of evidence now shows that while there are various pathways that contribute to the onset of chronic pain, the approaches to managing chronic pain difficulties are more similar than they are different. Research on chronic pain increasingly demonstrates that children with a wide range of pain-related conditions seem to suffer in similar ways. Not only do they struggle with persistent discomfort, but a majority of children with chronic pain also suffer from the same constellation of difficulties including sleep disruption, increased stress, challenges in keeping up with friends and activities, changes in mood, school-based difficulties, and more. These secondary problems are a big obstacle to overcoming chronic pain and part of the reason why the strategies presented in this book are appropriate for a wide range of pain-related experiences, including those related to pediatric diseases, such as

- Juvenile rheumatoid arthritis
- Endometriosis
- Irritable bowel disease
- Ehlers-Danlos syndrome
- Sickle cell anemia
- Cancer

and those that may emerge in non-disease-related situations, such as

- Post-injury pain
- Post-surgical pain
- Musculoskeletal pain
- Migraine headache

- Chronic daily headache
- Post-concussive headache
- Complex regional pain syndrome (also called reflexive sympathetic dystrophy)
- Fibromyalgia
- Postural orthostatic tachycardia syndrome
- Neuropathic pain
- Pain amplification syndrome
- Functional abdominal pain

My goal in writing this book is to help parents understand the often counterintuitive world of chronic pain in children, assist them in identifying underlying triggers or factors that may make their child's pain worse, and most importantly, arm them with the specific skills, strategies, information, and resources they need to increase comfort, reduce pain, and foster their child's adaptive growth and development.

This book is primarily about the psychological and behaviorally based strategies that are so important to the recovery from chronic pain. But it also includes information about common medications and supplements used in the treatment of chronic pain, an explanation of the role of physical and occupational therapy, and a review of alternative and complementary treatments. Understanding how all of these pain-management components are integrated into a comprehensive pain-management plan will help you and your child create a successful blueprint for his or her own recovery.

In order to present a comprehensive approach to easing the symptoms and side effects of chronic pain, I consulted with an army of professionals in and around the field of pain management, including pain-management physicians, gastrointestinal specialists, orthopedic specialists, sports medicine experts, neurologists, pediatricians, psychologists, social workers, physical therapists, nutritionists, acupuncturists, Reiki specialists, and others. This book represents the collective wisdom of many clinical providers who, like myself, work on the front lines every day to help alleviate symptoms associated with pediatric pain.

While interviewing and researching for this book, I came to recognize that most providers of pediatric pain services share a deeply held belief that there is both an art and science to the clinical practice of managing pediatric pain. I have grounded this book in the most up-to-date empirical science that has shaped the gold standard of practice in this clinical area. At the same time, it is my hope that this book also captures the essential art of pain management: an individualized approach to care that is deeply endowed with compassion, patience, human connection, and an unwavering commitment to the belief that things will almost certainly improve.

Acknowledgments

The success I've had in the field of pediatric pain management, which has led to the opportunity to write this book, is a debt that is owed to many. First and foremost, I am deeply indebted to all of my past and current patients for trusting me with their most challenging difficulties and placing their confidence in my care. I would never have had the knowledge or courage to write this book if I'd not been lucky enough to accompany so many inspiring families through the process of learning to manage chronic pain.

I am extremely grateful to Charles Berde, Chief of the Pain Treatment Service at Boston Children's Hospital. Dr. Berde's monumental contributions to the treatment of pediatric pain are continually inspiring and his ongoing passion for this field is contagious. Moreover, while it's easy for a department chair to applaud innovative work, it's much harder to provide the infrastructure to incubate fledgling ideas as Dr. Berde has repeatedly done on my behalf. With Neil Schechter, Director of the Chronic Pain Clinic at Boston Children's Hospital, I share a deep investment in teaching others what we have learned from our collective experiences in the field. Working collaboratively with him on a daily basis has been instrumental in shaping my career and I am grateful to him for his remarkable ability to treat me as a seasoned colleague while simultaneously providing invaluable mentorship at every turn.

I am also thankful to my colleague Deirdre Logan who recruited me to the Pain Treatment Service at Boston Children's Hospital ten years ago and has served as a compassionate friend, role model, and inspired leader. To my amazing psychology colleagues, Laura Simons, Karen Kaczynski, Christine Sieberg, Caitlyn Conroy, Rupa Gambhir, Edin Randall, and Allison Smith, I thank you all for your collaborative genius, professional support, and friendship. Working with this team of brilliant women is a driving force in my career. I am also grateful to all my collaborators in the Pain Treatment Service, especially my clinic-based colleagues Christine Greco, Susan Sager, Pradeep Dinakar, Luke Wang, Alyssa Lebel, and Navil Sethna and to my research assistant, Christina Iversen. I would never have set out on the path to write a book if not for the early support of two valued colleagues. I am thankful for the advice of Gerald Koocher, who convinced me that this was a book that needed to be written, and for the encouragement of Elisa Bronfman, who poked and prodded me through the early phases of this project and cheered me on through the middle and end.

A special and most sincere note of thanks goes to my talented collaborators in various disciplines who have read drafts of this manuscript and provided commentary that has at every step of the way made this a better book: Shannon O'Dell, Melinda Hogan, Peter Rafalli, Sam Nurko, Wendy Elverson, Rupa Ghambir, Deirdre Logan, Neil Schechter, Laura Simons, Lori Lazdowsky, Seetal Cheema, and Christine Greco.

I am also indebted to my graduate school mentor, Grayson Holmbeck, who set me on my professional path and continues to be one of my most trusted and respected colleagues. Many thanks to my loyal friends and colleagues who have helped me navigate the process of writing this book and cheered me on from near and far, especially Deborah Friedman, Jennifer Lebovidge, Sean Cashman, Elizabeth Keane, Nathalia Holt, Larkin Holt, Sarah Elliot, and Jill Rubenstein.

I am so grateful to my editor at the Yale University Press, Jean Thomson Black, for her persistent enthusiasm for this book, unwavering encouragement, and targeted advice. I'd like also to thank my copyeditor, Julie Carlson, for approaching my manuscript with the warmth of a parent, knowledge of a child development expert, and infinite flexibility.

Last, but most certainly never least, I wish to thank my family who know that none of this would have happened without their love, encouragement, and support. I thank my Dad, David Millstein, for gifting me with a love of writing and helping to cultivate my internal drive to find a way to make the world a better place. To my Mom, Nancy Millstein Marks, and my stepfather, Charles Marks, you have provided immeasurable support for each of my professional and personal endeavors; I am grateful to you both for all the ways, big and small, you have helped to foster my success. With her quick humor, listening ear, and daily dose of compassion, my "twin" sister Deborah Kronenberg is nothing less than everything a sister should be. Working together with her to balance the often-unbalanced world of professional pursuits and motherhood is a stabilizing force in my life. I am also grateful to the well of support I've had along the way from many other family members including Josh Kronenberg, Scott Millstein, Jae Lee, Joan Coakley, Chris Coakley, Liz Martin, Robert Liverman, and Helene Bernstein. And Nicole Henry, you are as much a part of our family as anyone. Thank you for the love and care you have for our family and for your graceful ability to keep us all afloat amidst the chaos.

To my amazing husband, Gerry, and two sons, Curran and Graham, this book is dedicated to you. Gerry, you are my rock and my sustaining force. Thank you for your unconditional love, for masterfully helping to keep everything on track while I worked full time and wrote a book, and for your impossibly gracious way of making me feel like superwoman even on my worst days. Curran, my son, you are wise beyond your nine years. Your life experiences have already taught you that medical stress is hard but that learning skills to cope with the stress and discomfort keeps you bouncing along. Your keen ability to soothe your mind and body will serve you well in all of your courageous endeavors and I am grateful that my education has helped me to help you in your times of need. Graham, at four years old you have thankfully yet to have pain beyond your skinned knees. Nevertheless, one day you will come to understand that as we practice gentle belly breaths at night while rocking together I am at once focused on breathing in your sweet smell and doing what little I can to prepare you for whatever challenges may come your way.

Part I

On Your Mark: Understanding What Pain Is (and Is Not)

The purpose of pain is to alert our body to danger and protect it from harm. If you slice your finger with a knife or touch a hot burner, your body produces a pain sensation known as *acute pain* so that you will quickly move away or get help. Treatment for injuries accompanied by acute pain usually follows a well-established, intuitive plan that might include cleaning the wound, getting stitches, taking pain medication, or resting the injured body part until it has healed. When the body has sufficiently healed, the acute pain sensations go away completely, letting you know that you can safely return to your regular daily routines.

Chronic or persistent pain, by contrast, is not straightforward. Chronic pain is not protective, not predictable, and not intuitive. This is a major reason why chronic pain is such a frustrating condition for kids and parents alike.

What is chronic pain, and why is it not protective? Chronic pain is defined by health professionals as any pain that persists for more than three months and can emerge from a variety of sources. Chronic pain can occur in any part of the body, but in pediatrics it most commonly includes chronic daily headaches, abdominal pain, musculoskeletal pain, and neuropathic (nerve) pain. Chronic pain can be associated with chronic health conditions such as arthritis, sickle cell disease, and irritable bowel disease, or can develop after an injury, surgery, or viral infection. What surprises many parents is that chronic pain can also emerge seemingly out of the blue. This is often the case for persistent pain problems, such as fibromyalgia, chronic daily headache, back pain, or functional abdominal pain.

In many cases chronic pain is more like a habit for the body than a warning of actual danger. I like to compare chronic or recurrent pain to a broken alarm clock. Imagine that your morning alarm clock goes off and you roll over to hit the snooze button, but it doesn't turn off like it's supposed to do. You try banging the snooze bar, switching the alarm off, unplugging the clock, taking out the batteries, and even throwing it out the window, but it still keeps ringing, even though you're fully awake. The pain alarm in our body can be just like this broken alarm clock. It can just keep ringing and ringing even though it's not helping in any way. In some cases, an illness, injury, or disease process sets off the ringing alarm of pain; in others, it's not clear what triggered it.

From a medical perspective, chronic pain can be a challenging problem to treat in part because there may initially be a lack of consensus on the underlying cause of the pain and how to treat it. In fact, one research study found that pediatricians could not agree on the cause of chronic pain in almost 60 percent of patients, and for a third of those patients, they could not agree on how to treat the symptoms. Because of this uncertainty, it can take weeks, months, or in some cases even years for families to really understand and treat their child's chronic pain problem. Even in the best-case scenarios, when the diagnostic process goes smoothly and a well-designed treatment plan is put into place, there are many factors that can influence how quickly and completely a child will recover.

Why some 25 percent of children will develop chronic pain and others will not is still unclear, though we are learning more about the risk and protective factors that may influence the onset of chronic pain. For example, we know that a family history of pain, early pain experiences, anxiety, depression, fear of pain, sensory sensitivities, and being female can all increase a child's vulnerability to chronic pain. We also know that staying active, feelings of self-efficacy, having supportive teachers in school, and maintaining positive peer relationships may be protective against the onset of chronic pain. Yet even with this increased generalized understanding, there is currently no effective way to predict which individuals will develop chronic pain, how long it will last, and who will have recurrent pain difficulties. Equally as frustrating is that once a chronic pain cycle begins, there is not a one-size-fits-all solution for the problem.

As parents we all rely on our intuitions to care for our children. These intuitions come from past experiences of successfully helping our children to recover from illness or injury. Chronic pain, however, follows a whole new set of rules, some of which are counterintuitive: for instance, rest is commonly viewed as being counterproductive to the recovery from chronic pain, and the simple act of checking in with children about their pain can lead to worsening symptoms. Managing chronic pain, then, requires a broad understanding of the mind-body relationship as well as knowledge about the role of the brain and nervous system in modulating the experiences of pain, pain-related stress, and mood.

The good news is that when parents can better understand the complexity of chronic pain, disability, and medical stress, they can begin to help "reset" the chronic pain alarm. The faster that parents and their kids can understand and implement effective strategies for the management of pain, the more quickly the healing can begin.

1

Beyond Intuition: Helping a Child Suffering from Chronic Pain

Many years ago, when my older son was sixteen months old, he had what appeared to be a fainting spell while sitting in his high chair having breakfast. He just slumped over and closed his eyes. After about three seconds, he woke up and seemed okay. But being a new mother, I was concerned, so I speed-dialed the pediatrician. She suggested simply keeping an eye on him to see if it happened again. About an hour later he was toddling along and suddenly slumped to the ground. He quickly stood right back up and continued playing as if nothing had happened. I shrugged it off thinking he just tripped on something I didn't see or was goofing around. But about an hour after that, while he was having his morning snack, he had a full-fledged tonic-clonic seizure: his eyes rolled back in his head, he gritted his teeth, and his little body stiffened and then started shaking. It lasted only a minute, but it was terrifying. My husband and I practically threw him in the car and rushed straight to the emergency room. By the time we got there, he seemed perfectly fine again.

We spent four hours in the emergency room with our child under observation, and the doctors could find nothing wrong with him. But just when we were meeting with the physician to discuss a plan for discharge, my son slumped on the exam table and had another seizure. This time it was longer and the shaking was more violent. The physician scooped up my stiff and seizing baby in his arms and ran down the halls of the emergency room, shouting a string of orders to nursing staff. Within minutes, my son was strapped to a stretcher with IV's in his arms and oxygen flowing. After what seemed like an eternity, he came out of the seizure screaming, crying, and thrashing. It was awful. My husband and I were both in tears. Our son immediately underwent a lumbar puncture, CT scan, and blood work. By the time we had finished in the emergency room we knew the problem wasn't a tumor or meningitis, but we didn't have a clue as to why he was having a flurry of seizures. He was admitted to the general pediatrics floor at around midnight. I was physically and emotionally exhausted.

When we had left the house to bring my son to the emergency room, I had a sense that it was going to be a long day, so I had quickly packed his pacifier, his favorite stuffed bear, and his favorite book, a pop-up book of jungle animals. I was just settling into the very uncomfortable chair in our room for the night when my son had another seizure. We screamed for the nurses. They called the doctors. We had a code red in our room within minutes. They shot my son full of medications but the seizure didn't stop. Doctors began talking in hushed tones about "status epilepticus," a very dangerous, sometimes life-threatening condition in which seizure activity cannot be disrupted. My son was in and out of consciousness and when he was not actively seizing he was crying hysterically. As the doctors were preparing my son for transfer to intensive care, one of the nurses came to my side and asked, "Is there anything you might try to help your son calm down a bit?"

I jumped into action.

I grabbed his favorite pop-up book, hopped up on his elevated bed, and began rapidly flipping through the pop-up pictures. "Look at this, look at this, it's your favorite book!" I said, trying to capture his attention and distract him from the many doctors surrounding his bed. But he just cried louder. I got closer to him, I put the pictures closer to his face thinking maybe his vision was off with all the seizure activity, and

I talked louder, thinking maybe he couldn't hear me over the buzzers, alarms, and shouting of orders going on around him. But he just kept crying.

Then the nurse gently tapped me on the shoulder and said, "Perhaps you could try quietly soothing him with his favorite lullaby?"

Oh. (Long, deep sigh.)

Yes, that did seem like a good idea.

And I did just what she suggested. I put the book down and quietly began singing his favorite lullaby in his ear. I don't know if he heard me, or if the powerful drugs he was given finally kicked in, but as I was singing, his little body relaxed and the seizures slowed.

When the situation had stabilized and I could finally catch my breath, I remember asking myself, "Why hadn't I thought of that?" Soft, quiet singing is what the moment had called for, and I often soothed him at home in this way. My loud demands for him to pay attention to his book and the bold jungle pop-up pictures seemed only to escalate the situation. I felt I had totally missed the boat. How could my first intuitions have been so wrong?

The really interesting part for me is that my son's nurse didn't know that I was a trained pediatric psychologist. She didn't know that I spend my working hours teaching children how to cope with pain and medical stress and teaching parents how to respond to their child's pain and stress. She knew only that I was a Mom—a Mom who was in crisis because my child was in crisis. So she knew I might not be thinking as clearly as I usually do. And she was right.

If I could have stepped outside this situation for a moment, I would have seen that flashing pop-up pictures of jungle animals in my son's face while trying to be louder than all the medical noise around him was pretty much the exact opposite of what was needed in that moment. I like to think of myself as an intuitive parent. I like to think that I know what my children need most, and that I give it to them. But when my son was so sick, I panicked and was only thinking, "I just need to get his attention away from everything going on around him." I was off my game, and my first intuition was not the best choice.

We spent several days in the ICU and thankfully, my son made a full recovery. But I think about this moment a lot when I work with my families who have a child in pain. It gives me great humility and great compassion for the challenge of helping parents who have a child in crisis. I know firsthand that when a child is in crisis, a parent is in crisis, too. I also know that as much as we like to think otherwise, parenting is not always intuitive. I believe that parents do know their children best, but when children are in pain, parents naturally feel panicked and desperate and under these challenging conditions, first intuitions are not always right.

Below are five of the most common "first intuitions" that parents have shared with me when they are coping with a child who has chronic pain and medical stress. Parents who respond with these first intuitions are trying to do what they feel is best for their child. But just like the nurse who tapped me on the shoulder to gently share that I should shift my approach, I often need to share with parents in crisis that they need to shift their approach, too.

"My child's pain and medical difficulties are real, so psychological strategies won't help."

Parents often tell me that their child's pain is a physical problem, not a psychological problem. They think that a referral to a psychologist somehow implies that the medical community thinks their child's pain is "in their head," or worse, that doctors don't even believe their child has "real" pain.

I wish I could say that doctors don't ever feel that way. But I've been in the field long enough to know that some families do have the unfortunate experience of having a physician directly or indirectly indicate that a child's pain is just a psychological problem. Usually the doctors who come to this conclusion can't clearly identify a cause for the persistent pain, or can't quickly fix the problem with surgery or medication. In their minds, that means that there is a psychological root to the pain.

This bias is why I am always careful to ensure that parents understand the value and benefit of psychological interventions for pain at the on-set of treatment. Over the past twenty years there has been a dramatic increase in research on chronic pain, which has led to the understand-ing that chronic pain can no longer be thought of as either physical or psychological. It is far more complex. Importantly, psychological strate-gies can help to reduce pain even when psychological problems are not the cause of the pain, in the same way that Tylenol can reduce fevers even though a lack of Tylenol is not the cause of the fever. Whether your child's pain emerged from an injury, disease, illness, or genetic disposi-tion, or came on out of the blue does not matter. Cognitive behavioral strategies that use the mind and body to target pain have become gold-standard treatments in the world of pain management for children.

"My child needs more rest."

When a child has strep throat or a sprained ankle, rest is of the utmost importance. In the counterintuitive world of chronic pain management, however, rest often exacerbates symptoms. Once pain transforms from a short-term problem to a longer-term problem, daytime rest and in-activity lead to deconditioning and changes in the autonomic nervous system. Both of these developments can lead to increased pain. Pro-longed rest can also lead to the onset of new pain problems and con-tribute to fatigue, insomnia, mental fogginess, and changes in mood. So while our first intuition tells us to let kids rest when they don't feel well, I'm going to explain in this book how and why kids often do far better with less rest and more activity.

"The more I do for my child, the faster she will recover."

When children experience pain, parents are drawn to care for them with extra love and attention. Parents who have a child with pain often help by taking over their child's chores, providing more homework as-sistance, bringing their child extra drinks or snacks, helping a child to get dressed, and generally pitching in wherever they feel they can do something, anything really, to make their child's life easier.

But once a pain problem has become chronic, sometimes the key to recovery is having parents do *less*. Children need to know that their parents have confidence in their ability to manage their own discomfort. When parents find ways to ease out of helping with daily tasks and activities, the message they send to their child is that they believe their child is well enough to do these things on his or her own.

This may seem like a subtle message, but it's a significant one. Within the research literature there is a term called "miscarried helping," which describes the downside of being too helpful for too long. Parents who adopt the day-to-day tasks that are developmentally appropriate for their child to do seem to unintentionally reinforce a child's belief that they are too sick, or too fragile, or too overwhelmed to do these things for themselves. On some level, kids think, "If Mom is actually making my bed and putting on my socks, I must really be in bad shape."

And while kids may initially be appreciative of very helpful parents, over time those same helping behaviors can actually lead to increased conflict in the parent-child relationship. It's a sticky cycle to undo. Parents *can* help their kids in very important ways, but they need to learn how to fight their intuition to do more caretaking of their child at every turn.

"I should always know how much pain my child is experiencing."

Our intuition as parents tells us to check in with our children frequently about their pain. This seems to make good sense. Of course, the medical community also reinforces this intuition. Any time you step foot in a doctor's office with a pain complaint, the first thing the doctor does is ask for a pain rating. Providers ask your child, "On a scale of 'zero' to 'ten,' with 'zero' meaning no pain at all, and 'ten' meaning the worst pain you could imagine, what number is your pain?"

I'll admit it—this is a clear-cut example of do what I say and not what I do. I myself collect pain ratings of my patients at almost every visit.

Most of my colleagues do the same. We include these ratings in a child's medical record and use them clinically to assess whether a patient has the subjective experience of feeling better. Some providers even request that parents or patients make a daily log of pain ratings over the course of a week or two to get a sense of the pattern of the pain.

Parents frequently adopt the zero-to-ten pain scale as a quick and easy way to learn how their child is feeling at any given moment. Some parents routinely spend a lot of time trying to obtain information about the severity and quality of a child's pain throughout the day, while other parents simply say, "What's your number?" Parents feel that this check-in communicates care, concern, and investment in their child. They also sincerely want to know how their child is doing. It certainly seems like a reasonable thing to ask.

All too often, however, this pain check-in becomes a habit for both kids and parents. Parents may ask for a pain rating when a child wakes up, after breakfast, while their child is watching TV, before their child takes medication, after their child takes medication, after a walk or a physical therapy session, before bed, and even in the middle of the night if a child wakes up with pain. Parents may also get in the habit of asking about pain when a child grimaces, sighs, seems to be having a bad day, or even seems to be having a particularly good day. Kids start to report this number to parents a lot as well. A child might say, "I'm not sure I can go to school, I'm a 'seven' today." This can seem like a pretty streamlined communication system, but all this talking about pain and pain ratings can backfire.

Research shows that the simple act of asking about pain leads to more pain. Every time children are asked for a pain rating, they have to stop what they're doing and think, "How badly do I hurt right now?" This attention to the pain is linked to an increase in pain. The less that children focus on their pain symptoms, the more they focus on other, more important things and the better they feel.

Pain ratings are entirely subjective and parents are urged to keep in mind that pain ratings alone do not reflect how well a child is doing. In other words a pain level of ten does not necessarily reflect maximum debilitation nor does it necessarily imply that there is a worsening medical course. It's counterintuitive, but it's verifiable and true. Kids who report feeling "ten" on the zero-to-ten pain scale can frequently go to school and be active with friends, while kids who rate their pain as five on the same scale may struggle to get to school and withdraw from friends and activities. There is frequently no association between pain rating and daily function. Many providers, then, feel that progress is best measured by how *functional* a child is, not how a child rates his or her pain.

So while pain ratings may be the most common way the medical community currently documents pain, it's far from a perfect system. Yes, I ask kids to rate their pain in my clinical work, but I don't put a lot of stock in the numbers and neither should parents. Parents need to learn how to break the habit of talking about pain and assessing pain levels at home. There are more helpful ways that parents can learn to communicate care and concern (see Chapter 4).

"It's not fair to expect my child to resume normal activities until his pain is gone."

It will not feel right at first to most parents, but it's true: frequent or persistent pain problems sometimes do not resolve until *after* kids are back in their routines. Indeed, getting back to routines is part of how we reset the pain alarm.

Dr. Neil Schechter, one of my colleagues, frequently explains to patients that persistent pain is like a software problem. When a computer freezes or crashes, it's almost always due to a software error. He explains that if you peeked inside the computer you wouldn't see anything wrong with the computer hardware (wires, filaments, microchips). The same is true for the body in the case of chronic pain. There is nothing wrong with the hardware (bones, muscles, organs), but the software that sends messages throughout the nervous system is on the fritz. How do you reboot the software to get rid of the chronic pain? One important step is to feed the malfunctioning nerves "normal data." Nerves need to be exposed to regular, normal input to reset. Once they continuously get the message that regular activities are not inherently harmful, they start to restore themselves. For this reason, increasing a child's daily functioning at home and school is one of the *first* steps in managing pain. The key is to do this gradually so that the child feels empowered, not overwhelmed (see Part 4).

Second Intuitions

As parents, we often act with our hearts first and our minds second. When our kids are sick or in crisis we do what we think is best, and we should never have a moment's regret about that noble impulse. But being open to suggestions and trying new things is also a part of good parenting. For this reason, I hope this book will be just like the caring nurse who tapped me on the shoulder to suggest I change my approach when my son was sick. Honestly, her advice was hard to hear at first. After all, I know my child better than she ever would. But that nurse did have special knowledge: she knew what children with seizures needed most from their parents. It was new to me and that's in part why it felt so scary.

The management of persistent pain and prolonged medical stress is not intuitive. But parents play a very important role in the process and they already have in hand many of the skills they need to help their child. With good information and structured guidance, parents can learn how to abandon those first intuitions that are not helpful and instead adopt new strategies that will help them to support their child more effectively.

♦

How to Help

1. EVALUATE YOUR OWN PARENTING PRACTICES

If your child is struggling with chronic or recurrent pain, consider that some of the first intuitions you have about how to help your child may not be working. It's easy to get off track when your child is hurting or when there has been a long and potentially confusing medical course. By carefully evaluating your parenting practices, you may begin to identify places where your first intuitions have become less well suited for your child's recovery. Parents must be very involved in their child's lives when chronic pain is an ongoing concern. But it's important to be involved in the right ways. Learning the adaptive parenting strategies that lead to increased comfort and function, and abandoning the parenting practices that are known to reinforce pain cycles, is critical.

2. STAY OPEN TO NEW IDEAS

Every family is different and every child in pain has unique challenges. This book presents numerous strategies for helping to ease pain and improve well-being and I encourage you to approach each idea with an open mind. Some strategies will work well right from the start, some will work only after several weeks of consistent practice, and still others might not be a great fit for you or your child. I encourage all parents to try a variety of new strategies and to keep in mind that some of the best ones in the long run may appear to have only a small effect at first. Parents should expect that if their child has been in chronic pain for months or years, the success of new ideas and strategies may not be clearly evident right from the start.

3. MOVE FORWARD

Managing chronic pain can be a major challenge. If you've fallen into any of the first intuition traps, rest assured you are in good company. Keep in mind that it's easy to pick out a few things that any parent could do better, but it would usually take years to make a list of everything parents do right. For this reason I tell parents not to waste a second on feelings of frustration or self-blame and instead direct their energies toward thinking about the positive changes they can make going forward.

2

The Science of Pain and the Mind-Body Connection

Clearly the mind and the body are connected. The physical evidence is unmistakable. Yet the prevailing wisdom for centuries was that the mind had nothing to do with the body, or for that matter, with the sensation of pain. Thankfully we are more enlightened today. The obvious connection between the mind and the body is not only accepted, but foundational to much of what modern medicine offers.

Still, skeptics exist. If you're on the fence about the mind-body connection, you are in good company. In fact, the majority of people I meet don't fully "buy in" to the mind-body connection, or if they do, they don't fully appreciate its significance to pain management. Yet consider this evidence:

- More than 85 percent of people who have an amputated limb experience pain in that missing limb.
- People recovering from surgery who have plants in their hospital rooms report experiencing less pain than do patients who do not have plants in their rooms.
- Neuroimaging studies confirm that when patients believe that placebos (sugar pills) contain pain-reducing medications they not only

report reduced pain, but also have decreased activity in the areas of the brain and spinal cord responsible for processing pain signals.

In these examples, it's impossible to ignore the role of the mind in pain sensation. Indeed the mind, or more technically the brain, controls everyone's perception of pain all of the time. The brain piece of the pain puzzle is precisely why there is never a one-to-one correspondence between the severity of an illness or injury and the sensation of pain. It also explains why the severity of an illness, injury, or pain does not directly relate to how much a person can do or how well a person functions in his or her life. The key to unraveling these seemingly confusing relationships lies entirely in our understanding of how pain is processed in the brain. This knowledge informs many of our most important interventions for children struggling with pain.

The Brain and Nervous System

Here's a quick anatomy lesson that will help you to understand the important relationship between the brain, the nervous system, and pain. The brain houses the biggest collection of nerves in our body and thus is thought of as the boss of our entire nervous system. Next in command is the spinal cord. Together the brain and spinal cord form the central nervous system; essentially the headquarters for the human body. Beyond the central nervous system is the peripheral nervous system, which is made up of the somatic and the autonomic nervous systems. Both of these systems send and receive messages to the spinal cord and brain, but each system has its own very specific job description. The somatic system employs sensory nerves to communicate messages about how we sense the world around us. For example, sensory nerves send messages to our brain about what's hot or cold, what's soft or rough, what smells good and what stinks, and importantly, what hurts and what doesn't. The autonomic nervous system is responsible for sending messages about much of what we do that we don't usually think about, such as keeping our heart beating continuously and ensuring that we blink approximately twenty-five thousand times per day. The

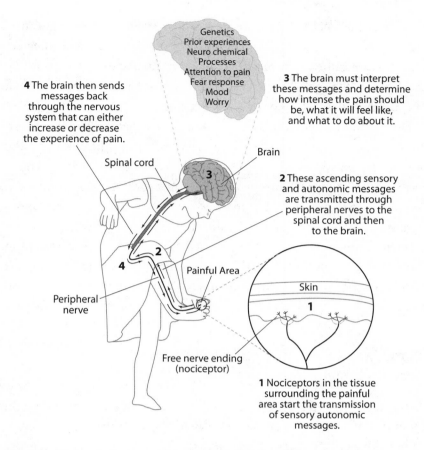

4 The brain then sends messages back through the nervous system that can either increase or decrease the experience of pain.

Genetics
Prior experiences
Neuro chemical
Processes
Attention to pain
Fear response
Mood
Worry

3 The brain must interpret these messages and determine how intense the pain should be, what it will feel like, and what to do about it.

Brain

Spinal cord

2 These ascending sensory and autonomic messages are transmitted through peripheral nerves to the spinal cord and then to the brain.

Painful Area

Skin

Peripheral nerve

Free nerve ending (nociceptor)

1 Nociceptors in the tissue surrounding the painful area start the transmission of sensory autonomic messages.

How the human body senses, interprets, and responds to pain.

autonomic nervous system also sends the messages that regulate the stress response known as "fight or flight," a defense system that is frequently implicated in pain processing.

Consider what happens throughout your nervous system when you stub your toe. Pain receptors in your toe, called nociceptors, send sensory and autonomic signals through the peripheral nerves in your foot and leg to the spinal cord and then into the brain. Once there, the signal activates a response team to form a sort of injury report. It must answer these questions: What happened? What needs to be done? And importantly, how much does this need to hurt? The answers to these questions determine whether the pain ebbs or is felt more intensely.

Usually the nociceptors in the toe will continue to send pain messages to the brain until the skin, tissues, or bones are sufficiently healed. But sometimes the nervous system can continue to send signals to the brain indicating that the toe is still hurt, even when the toe is healed. This is how a chronic pain cycle can get started.

How could our nervous system make this mistake? The central nervous system is flooded with incoming messages all the time and the brain must constantly interpret signals and decide how, when, where, and what to do in response to all these messages. To help in this endeavor, the pain processing centers of the brain routinely solicit input from the memory and emotion centers of the brain so that they can put the incoming pain (nociceptor) messages from the nervous system in context. Past experiences, made up of memories and emotions, in part help to determine the frequency, intensity, and duration of the pain sensation.

Memory and Emotions Help to Decode Nervous Systems Messages

Pain is a sensory sensation produced by the brain via nervous system communications. In many ways, it functions like other sensory communications within our nervous system. For example, when sensory nerves in the nose send messages to the brain indicating that it has detected the scent of a cake baking in the oven, this message is processed with input from the memory and emotion centers of the brain. If one's past experiences with cake are pleasant (delicious taste, a fun party, a sugar rush), the brain and central nervous system might send a message to the motor nerves in the face to produce a smile and might release the hormone serotonin, which generates happy feelings. Without a positive past memory of cake, the brain would not send out a signal to smile and would not release mood-boosting neurotransmitters. Without context, the signal would just be a signal. Your brain might process the scent, but there would be no positive response and no positive reaction.

If we don't have a collection of past memories to rely on, the brain tries its best to make the right assessment, but this can be a difficult task. For example, many young children are afraid of loud noises. My own children, too, went through a phase at about age two where they would stop everything they were doing and run over to me in a state of panic every time a neighbor turned on a lawnmower. Interestingly, until my children would bring the noise to my attention, I wouldn't have even noticed the sound of the lawnmower. It's so common for me to hear a lawnmower that my brain doesn't even register the sound. For sure my auditory nervous system sends messages to my brain saying something like, "There is a loud noise outside your home." But since I have heard thousands of lawnmowers before, my brain simply responds, "Don't worry, no need to react, that's just a lawnmower." Although I hardly seemed to notice the sound at all, it was quite different for my young children. When their brain received the sensory information "There is a loud noise outside your home," their young brains responded with "Oh my gosh! That could be really bad! Take cover, get Mommy!" For my children, this sensory input (loud noise) triggered an emotional response (fear), motor response (run to Mommy), and an autonomic nervous system response (racing heart, shortness of breath, shaking). Of course, over time, after hearing many lawnmowers and, importantly, after seeing that I wasn't the least bit alarmed when the lawnmower turned on, my children learned that they didn't need to take cover each time a lawnmower was started. The positive, nonthreatening experiences of lawnmowers influenced their nervous system signals so that they felt much less fearful. At this point they could experience the sound without distress and without interrupting their activities.

Incoming sensory signals, whether they are olfactory (cake baking), auditory (lawnmower), or pain-based, are all interpreted with help from the memory and emotion centers of the brain. Part of managing chronic pain is understanding how memories and emotions universally influence the sensation of pain and learning to modify these aspects of pain processing. This is hard work. Unlike my young boys who quickly adapted to the lawnmower noise because there were no adverse experiences linked to the noise, pain is consistently an adverse experience and repeated pain experiences can form negative habit loops that are hard to break.

Pain as a Habit

Many pain researchers have come to think of chronic pain as a habit for the body. When the sensory signals that trigger the sensation of pain persistently flood the nervous system, the neural pathways that transmit these signals get a lot of traffic and adapt accordingly. At the start of a pain problem, these neural pathways may be like dirt roads through a wooded countryside. The signals can find their way through, but it takes a bit of effort. Over time, however, these pathways can become like well-traveled eight-lane superhighways that make it much easier and faster for signals to get through to the brain. The routine behaviors that kids develop in response to persistent pain can be thought of as habits, too. Napping or resting during the day, not going to school, reductions in general activity levels, being less involved with friends, sleeplessness, and poor study or work routines can all become habits for the body. Negative thinking patterns that develop in response to pain are also habit forming. Our brain can get in a rut or routine of interpreting pain as being awful and disabling, which can perpetuate more pain and lead to even more nervous-system sensitivity. Chronic pain habits for the body can become established over just a few weeks, but more often it takes a few months or years. And, it seems, the longer these habit loops have been in place, the harder they are to modify. One of our primary goals in pain management is to undo the habit loops that are known to maintain chronic pain cycles and replace them with more adaptive habits that can foster long-term comfort and reduce the sensation of pain.

Sensitization and Amplification

Habit loops would be hard enough to break if they were static. But it seems that without intervention, pain-related habits and pain sensations become more entrenched over time. This means that instead of adapting and getting used to the experience of pain, the body can become more sensitive to pain and more debilitated by the symptoms. The sensitization of the nervous system can cause a person to experience pain far beyond what would be expected given a particular illness or injury, or even when there is no clear underlying cause. Here's an example of how it works: Imagine that you had a slow drip in the faucet of a bathroom right outside your bedroom. At first, you might not notice it at all, but once you had tuned into the drip . . . drip . . . drip, you would probably find it pretty annoying. If every night you had to hear it, and no matter what you did it didn't stop, this relatively little problem would probably become very frustrating and eventually cause a lot of distress. You might even get to the point where all you seemed to hear every night was drip . . . drip . . . drip. Your auditory processing centers would become highly sensitized to this dripping sound and you might even start to hear it from other parts of the house. Even after you finally repaired the faucet, you may be amazed (and quite frustrated) to find that when you went to sleep you could swear you still heard drip . . . drip . . . drip.

This is an example of how a sensory signal can be amplified. What started as a small drip became a major problem because the auditory nervous system quickly became sensitized to the sound and in part because this signal was likely paired with negative interpretations ("Why won't this ever stop dripping!," "This is driving me crazy!").

In the case of chronic pain, the sensory nervous system can become highly attuned to a pain problem and thus, like ears sensitizing to the drip, become sensitized to the pain—to the point where all sorts of nervous system inputs start to be interpreted by the brain as painful. For example, in some cases light touch or vibrations can become excruciating for a person with sensitized nerves in an arm or leg, and minor bloating can be very painful for a child with sensitized abdominal nerves.

It is also possible to experience more widespread sensitization, called "central sensitization." This is when sensitivity that started in the peripheral nervous system begins to encompass the central nervous system (brain and spinal cord) as well. The process of central sensitization explains how it is possible (and not uncommon) for pain to spread from one part of the body to another. For example, a child with persistent nerve pain in a foot may find that the pain spreads up his or her leg or even "jumps" over to the other foot. A child with persistent abdominal pain may develop persistent headaches as well. A child with chronic back pain may develop widespread pain or symptoms of fibromyalgia. If spreading pain isn't bad enough, central sensitization may also be implicated in mood sensitivity; children may become more irritable, tearful, or anxious when their central nervous systems are sensitized.

If you think about chronic pain like a car alarm, you can start to understand that there can be a lot of variability in the sensitivity of individual nervous systems. Car alarms are designed to go off when there is actually someone breaking into a car. But sometimes car alarms go off when a car is lightly bumped, when a large truck passes by, or even seemingly out of the blue. When the alarm goes off and there is no threat of danger, it's considered a false alarm. Because chronic pain is by definition a pain that persists when there is no acute danger, it's often thought of as a false alarm as well. Why some car alarms are highly sensitive and others are not might be due to a variety of reasons such as manufacturing differences, electrical malfunctions, or other factors. Similarly, chronic pain and nervous system sensitivity are likely due to a variety of individual factors. Whatever the reason, the goal with an overly sensitive alarm—whether a car alarm or pain alarm—is to figure out how to recalibrate it.

◆

How to Help

1. TELL YOUR CHILD HOW THE NERVOUS SYSTEM WORKS

Explain to your child that the nervous system can become highly sensitive to pain and that the brain can begin to habitually focus on the pain, which can lead to feeling worse. Explain the mind-body connection to your child in a way that makes sense to both of you, and use examples of how the mind and body are connected:

Feeling happy when you smell a cake baking
Feeling relaxed when you touch a pet's soft fur
Feeling soothed when someone gently rubs your back
Feeling exhilarated after you go for a good run
Feeling your mouth water when you think about biting into a sour lemon

Explain that using mind-based strategies to manage pain can be a huge help and can reverse some of the sensitivity of the nervous system. Be sure to let your child know that using these mind-based strategies in no way implies that the pain is in his or her head or that the pain is not real pain.

2. CONSIDER YOUR CHILD'S MEMORIES AND PAST EXPERIENCES OF PAIN

Pain is frequently linked to negative memories and fears, and these emotions and memories need to be addressed. You might try talking together with your child about pain-related experiences or memories that may have been fearful, worrisome, or upsetting and explaining to your child that these can be responsible in part for the persistent nature of pain. There are many suggestions for exploring and managing negative feelings and memories in Chapter 4. If you think negative memories or experiences (especially traumatic experiences related to an injury or medical course) may be playing a role, but are not sure how to approach this issue, it may be worthwhile to consider an evaluation by a psychologist who specializes in pain management (see Chapter 6).

3. ANALYZE YOUR CHILD'S HABITS

What new habits have been formed since your child developed chronic pain? While you might have previously thought of routines like resting on the couch watching TV, going to school less, or sleeping late as ways of alleviating pain, consider that they might be pain-related habits that are contributing to your child's pain sensitivity. While habits like these may seem soothing, especially in the short term, there are other, more helpful ways to generate comfort that can help with the long-term goals for recovery (see Chapter 5).

4. ASK YOUR CHILD'S PHYSICIAN ABOUT THE POSSIBILITY OF SENSITIZATION OR CENTRAL SENSITIZATION

Sensitization to pain is a big problem for people who struggle with chronic pain. If you think your child is becoming very sensitive to sensations of light touch or has spreading pain, be sure to discuss this with your child's doctor. There are some medications that may help, and they can work well when coupled with the cognitive and behavioral strategies in this book. There are also physical therapy approaches that can be enormously helpful for reducing sensitization (see Chapter 7).

3

The Unavoidable Link between Pain and Stress

I've never met a child with pain or ongoing medical difficulties who does not also have stress, even if she is very good at hiding or downplaying it. Indeed, stress is an inherent part of pain. The pathway between pain and stress has often been described as bidirectional, meaning that pain causes stress, and stress causes pain. A thorough understanding of the relationship between pain and stress is part of the foundation for successful pain management.

Pain Causes Stress

Pain is such a negative and stressful sensory experience that we are biologically programmed to avoid it at all costs. Ensuring that we avoid pain is part of how we maintain our survival. So experiencing pain, or sometimes even anticipating pain, causes a cascade of biochemical responses in the body that generate a state of physical and emotional tension, also known as stress. This stress response is intended to help keep us safe.

Imagine for a moment that you are walking briskly down the sidewalk on a lovely spring day on your way to a favorite restaurant. Now envision the tip of your toe catching in a deep crack of the sidewalk. The instant you begin to trip forward, a biochemical stress response (also called the "fight or flight" response) is triggered. You feel a strong and immediate sense of fear and danger, your eyes dilate, your heart races, you draw a quick shallow breath, the small hairs on the back of your neck stand on end, and the muscles in your arms and legs automatically and instantaneously stiffen to brace you for the fall. After you hit the ground, you must do a quick appraisal of the situation to assess if you are hurt; and if so, where and how badly. Do you need medical care? Can you walk?

If you determine that you are okay, the stress response begins to subside. Your heart slows down, your muscles relax, your respiration returns to normal, and you slowly get up. If you realize that you're *not* okay, however, your body stays in a state of high physiological arousal or stress. Your heart keeps pumping fast, your breath remains short, your mind races and is highly vigilant, your muscles stay tight, your immune system is temporarily bolstered, your adrenaline is pumping, and though you may be aware that you are injured, it's possible you may not yet feel pain. This stress response is one of our best defenses. We don't think about it—it's a reflexive response, part of our autonomic nervous system that serves us well when we are faced with an acute or sudden injury like a fall.

Some features of this stress response serve us well in the long term, too. If you broke your ankle in that fall, you might be reluctant or even somewhat fearful to walk down that stretch of sidewalk again. To remind you to avoid experiencing this injury again, your body may produce an anticipatory fear or stress response. You might experience physical reactions similar to those that occurred the first time you tripped, though they may be less intense. This adrenaline-based, reflexive, and protective stress response can protect us when we're faced with painful or even potentially painful situations.

Interestingly, pain and stress are so intricately tied together that it can actually be very difficult to tease apart the fear and stress associated with pain and the sensory experience of pain itself. In its evolutionary wisdom, our brain has learned to store this information together in a single protective memory. Biologically, the pairing of the fear and stress response with the sensation of pain makes perfect sense because we need to avoid those things that cause us pain. But it can also do more harm than good. When pain is persistent, it commonly does not reflect a new threat to the body. Moreover, as an offshoot of our protective pain avoidance mechanisms, some people develop a persistent fear or stress response to chronic pain. As discussed in Chapter 1, the link between fear, stress, and chronic pain can become an unwelcome habit for the body.

Pain-Related Fear and Stress

Laura Simons, one of my psychologist colleagues at the Pain Treatment Service, studies the "fear of pain" response. The cycle works like this: a child experiences pain in a situation, becomes fearful of having more pain in that situation, and thus avoids any activity that he or she perceives as a trigger for pain. Avoidance might start with a very particular situation and then generalize to others. For example, if a child injured her knee while running down stairs, she might initially fear and avoid stairs, then she might start to worry that walking on any uneven surface might cause pain and start to avoid uneven surfaces, and then she might start to fear that walking on any surface could make her knee hurt and so decide to stop walking altogether. A fear of pain can develop for non-injury-related pain as well. For example, a child with chronic abdominal pain who experiences discomfort while at school may develop a fear of having pain in school, and so try to avoid attending school altogether.

Fear of pain causes overactivity in the autonomic nervous system, which in turn leads to other biological changes in the body. People who fear pain may feel on high alert, have stiff or rigid muscles, be more sensitive and reactive to pain, and be more protective of their bodies. All of these responses occur without conscious effort, but they are exhausting and a major source of pain-related stress for the body.

Reducing Pain-Related Fear and Stress

Some night when you're with your child, go into your bathroom together, close the door, and after telling your child what will happen next, turn out the lights. At first you probably won't be able to see a thing. But be patient. Within a few minutes, your eyes will adjust. First you'll start to make out the outline of objects. Then you'll start to see variations in color. Within a few minutes you'll most likely be able to see well enough to do a simple task such as washing your hands. But if when you first turned out the lights you had given up and turned the lights back on, convinced that you would never be able to see anything without them, your eyes would not have been exposed long enough to the dark to adapt. This "exposure" principle is a key concept for reducing the fear and stress associated with pain.

Think back to our example of falling on the sidewalk. Let's say that you needed to walk over that crack to get to your favorite restaurant every morning. The first time you walked over the crack again you'd likely feel stressed and recall the injury you had. The second and third times you'd likely also feel some stress. But over time, your body would learn that there is little danger in walking over the crack, and your stress response would subside. Working through the fear by trying again, and giving the body new, more reassuring, information, is a tried and true way to override the fear and stress response.

Once a doctor has medically cleared a child for activity, reducing the stress and fear associated with normal activities is an important goal. Starting small is essential. So, for example, the child who injured her knee and stopped walking might have the goal of taking just three steps while using a coping skill such as deep breathing and registering the positive idea, "Even if this hurts for a little while, it will help me to heal."

A child with irritable bowel syndrome who has developed a stress response to school can similarly learn to override this association by slowly increasing her time spent at school and managing any discomfort while there. If a child always returns home or abandons an activity when there is discomfort, she will never realize that her pain can be managed. This missed learning opportunity fuels increased stress and perpetuates pain cycles. Learning how to properly scaffold a child's return to activity and thereby reducing pain-related stress is discussed in Chapter 15.

Stress Causes Pain

Stress is not inherently a bad thing. When stress occurs once in a while, it can be very useful in our lives. Small to moderate amounts of stress produce adrenaline, a hormone that can increase productivity, boost our immune systems, afford us the ability to temporarily function on less sleep and less food, and generate feelings of wellness. Unfortunately, an enormous amount of research clearly demonstrates that when stress is continuous, it backfires on our systems. Too much adrenaline causes the release of the stress hormone cortisol and over time, this combination interferes with sleep cycles, depletes our immune response, creates feelings of uneasiness, produces chronic muscle tension, and can be a major contributing and maintaining factor in chronic pain cycles.

A stress response can be triggered by any event or situation that requires a high level of emotional or physical adaptation. If the stress is short-lived and the body has time to recover between stress responses, then it usually does not cause any ill effects. When stress is persistent, however, it takes a biological toll on the body.

As discussed earlier, pain and the fear of pain have been clearly identified as triggers for stress. But many other things cause stress as well. Some stressors are readily evident to most parents, such as bullying, divorce, and the loss of family members or pets. Yet other stressors are equally as important and often overlooked. Consider for a moment that the United States President's Council on Fitness, Sports & Nutrition states that in 2013 only one in three children has dedicated time for physical activity each day, while on average children spend about seven hours per day in front of a screen (TV, computer, video game, smartphone) and consume 40 percent of their calories from sugars and fats.

While parents may not routinely think about poor nutrition or inactivity as a source of stress, they are in fact biologically stressful.

Children and adolescents may also experience stress when cognitive or emotional demands in their environment exceed their developmental capabilities. For example, ubiquitous exposure to technology and media that are age-inappropriate can lead to significant stress because it can cause children to be confronted with images or issues that they are not emotionally equipped to manage. Similarly, when schools must practice lockdown drills and discuss terrorism or violence in schools, kids may experience this as a source of chronic emotional stress.

Children who are over-committed or overscheduled also commonly experience a high level of chronic stress. During my evaluations I routinely ask kids to tell me about their typical day. If the description includes getting home from school and practicing flute for an hour, then eating dinner on the fly in the back seat of the car while putting on cleats for soccer practice, then babysitting at the neighbor's house for an hour, then doing homework until 10:00 p.m., showering, and preparing for the SAT until 11:30 p.m., there is a stress problem. Parents may earnestly defend their child, saying, "I told her she's doing too much, but she really loves being in the band, playing soccer, and babysitting, and of course she has to prepare for the SAT."

It's wonderful when kids are busy and have time to pursue their interests and passions. But overloaded schedules are inherently stressful to most children and can impair their physical health. Ironically, parents and kids sometimes strive to get rid of pain symptoms so that all of the child's activities can resume without even recognizing that overpacked schedules or unrealistic expectations may be a trigger for pain. In these situations I ask parents to step in to help their child curtail some activities and so restore some balance to their routines. When children have the time they need to sit down for meals, have a quiet time before bed, and get to sleep at a reasonable hour, they often start to feel at least somewhat better.

Sometimes sources of stress can be hidden because they are viewed as a positive experience. For example, a family move may be a positive change for everyone in the family, but is also an inherently stressful experience for a child. Parents should also consider that the stress associated with a seemingly temporary, normative, and relatively minor incident such as a breakup with a boyfriend or girlfriend, can have lasting effects for an adolescent. Sources of stress can also sometimes fly under the radar. For example, I routinely ask parents to consider how academic pressure may contribute to a child's experience of stress. Parents often deny that they pressure their child to do well in school ("he wanted to take all honors classes; it was his idea"), failing to recognize that when the culture of the family conveys implicit goals for top-tier college entry and when scholastic achievement is consistently rewarded with high levels of parent praise and attention, the academic stress from parents can unknowingly be significant.

There is solid medical research to support the link between persistent daily stress and chronic pain conditions such as headache, back pain, chest pain, gastrointestinal disorders, chronic fatigue, temporomandibular joint (TMJ) disorder, limb pain, and other health problems. In some cases persistent stress is the underlying cause of the pain. But most commonly, something else—such as an injury, virus, or disease—triggered the pain and the stress response serves a supporting or maintaining role in the chronic pain cycle.

A Vicious Cycle

As I mentioned, many people think of stress and pain as a bidirectional type of process: pain causes stress and stress causes pain. I tend to think of pain and stress more like an insidious loop. The stress response uses an enormous amount of energy in our body. If the stress response is frequently triggered by pain or other sources of stress, the body becomes depleted and more problems emerge. The combination of chronic or recurrent pain and stress is associated with disruptions in sleep, appetite, mood, anxiety, memory, and learning. Moreover, the insidious pain and stress cycle can lead to neurochemical changes that make the body even more sensitive to pain, further exacerbating a child's distress.

Take for example Rebecca, a fourteen-year-old patient of mine who came in for treatment with burning, stabbing pain in her right foot. She had been on crutches for six months, and her pain had been diagnosed as complex regional pain syndrome (CRPS), a neuropathic pain condition that is frequently triggered by a minor injury. Rebecca openly discussed how her pain was getting in the way of her normal activities. She had fallen behind in school in part because she had so many doctor appointments and in part because some days she felt the pain made it too difficult to concentrate. She used to love school but after missing so many days she was afraid to go, worried that there would be tests or projects for which she was not well prepared. She had to stop playing softball and reported that she was frustrated about getting out of shape and about hardly ever seeing her teammates.

Rebecca's parents reported that Rebecca had high levels of pain, but denied that she was under any stress. They were a highly supportive family and recognized that Rebecca was struggling, but they failed to understand that the stress associated both with the pain and with the secondary problems that had emerged was playing a significant role in Rebecca's pain and related disability. Six months of foot pain, disruptions to school, a lack of physical activity, poor sleep, and missed opportunities to see teammates and friends would lead anyone to feel stressed. And for an adolescent who has the developmental goal of being more independent, it can be inherently stressful to be unable to walk without the use of crutches and to have to rely on others for help with daily tasks.

When we acknowledge that stress contributes to pain, we are in no way implying that a child's pain is an emotionally based problem. The biological connection between pain and stress is well established, and one of the best things parents can do is to openly embrace the fact that pain and stress are intricately related. Knowing this can itself open a pathway to healing. That is, although we may not be able to directly modify the underlying biological root of the pain—for example, the disease-related pain may persist, or an injury may take weeks more to heal—those biological triggers for pain are only part of the story. The stress responses that can trigger and exacerbate pain are equally important in the experience of pain. And everyone, regardless of their diagnosis, can learn adaptive ways to manage stress.

Beyond Pain, What Causes Persistent Stress for Your Child?

The first step in learning how to manage stress is figuring out what causes stress for *your* child. Persistent stress can come from many sources. Sources of stress for children can include, among many other things, major life events (divorce, loss of a family member or pet, moving to a new home), social difficulties (feeling left out or being teased in school), cultural factors (media over-exposure, high-stress academics, overloaded schedules (not enough time for meals and sleep), unhealthy eating habits (too much caffeine, sugary snacks, or energy drinks, eating too little or having irregular meals), uncomfortable environments (persistent noise, bright lights, lack of privacy), conflict within the home (arguing with parents, parental conflict, sibling rivalries), perfectionistic personality traits (working too hard to please others, setting unrealistic expectations), and even thinking negatively (self-critical thoughts, feeling unable to cope or hopeless, or feeling blamed or at fault).

Identifying what causes tension in your child's life can help you to make a plan for how to reduce stress. Some sources of stress such as noise problems, busy schedules, or sibling rivalries might be fairly easy to address. Others, like the loss of a loved one, long-standing academic challenges, or perfectionistic personality traits, are harder to change. In these cases, parents need to help their children find ways to bolster their self-care and coping skills to offset or reduce the effects of stress. Interventions might include building in extra time each day to do an activity your child truly enjoys, such as painting, reading, cooking, or playing a game. Teaching your child the relaxation skills in Part 3 are also a proven way to reduce the impact of stress.

Additionally, parents are encouraged to think carefully and critically about whether their own behaviors may be increasing a child's stress. For example, if your morning routines involve a lot of yelling and chaos because your child does not have his homework in his backpack, lunch packed, and teeth brushed, consider what you as a parent can do to help set a calmer tone. Though it may take extra effort to help your child assemble school materials the night before, or to create a child-friendly list or chart to guide the morning routines, it may be worthwhile to reduce everyone's stress. If you have an older adolescent, brainstorm together about which parts of the day or week feel most stressful and come up with a plan for making those times go more smoothly.

♦

How to Help

1. EXPLAIN THE LINK BETWEEN PAIN AND STRESS TO YOUR CHILD

Having a conversation with your child about the connection between pain and stress is vitally important. You might say something like "Our bodies are pretty amazing. We have a built-in stress response that is designed to protect us from pain and that is automatically triggered by pain, even without our knowing. This stress response may have been helpful when you first had pain, but now that your pain has been going on a long time, we want to manage the stress response. Retraining your body in this way will help you to feel better overall." Make sure your child understands that reducing stress helps with pain, but this does not take away from the physical reality of the pain: your child's pain is not just the result of feeling stressed.

2. TEACH YOUR CHILD HOW TO REVERSE THE FEAR OF PAIN

The fear of pain is a natural and protective stress response. When kids have chronic or persistent pain, however, they need to learn how to override the fear that can accompany pain and pain-related disability. If your child worries about experiencing pain in a particular situation, make a plan to help expose your child to that feared situation, little by little, in a gradually increasing way. Imagine that each exposure is like a rung on a ladder. With each step up the ladder your child progresses toward the goal of being able to tolerate the feared experience. For example, an adolescent whose doctor says he can become more physically active, but is afraid it might be painful, could take a five-minute walk with a pet or a friend as a first step, with running a full mile the ultimate goal. See Part 4 for suggestions on how to design a step-by-step plan for returning to these and other activities.

3. IDENTIFY TRIGGERS FOR STRESS AND PAIN

Keep a record for a few days of when your child appears to experience the most pain. What happened right before? What was going on around your child at the time? If you can identify certain situations, topics of conversation, or times of day that are associated with increased pain or pain-related stress, those can become targets for intervention. For example, if your child gets a headache everyday in math class, try to figure out what might be stressful during that time of day. Is your child confused in class? Overly hungry at that time of day? Annoyed by a classmate? Worried about homework? All of these potential triggers can be a source of stress and a trigger for pain.

4. REDUCE SOURCES OF STRESS

While isolating children from all stress is neither a feasible nor an adaptive goal, it can be helpful to think about what areas of your child's day or week might be unnecessarily stressful and work with your child to lighten the load, emotionally and physically. Chronic sources of stress such as overly busy schedules, academic pressures, poor nutrition, and a lack of physical activity can all be targets for intervention (see Part 4).

5. MONITOR YOUR OWN STRESS-BASED THOUGHTS AND ACTIONS

Children are very perceptive, and they tend to feel responsible and deeply concerned about problems that their loved ones are experiencing. It's especially important, then, to think about how your own stress response (over, for example, missed work, caring for other children and juggling other family responsibilities, frustration with teachers or doctors, and so on) may contribute to the stress of your child. Model those stress-management strategies you believe would help your child.

6. CONSIDER WORKING WITH A BEHAVIORAL HEALTH PROVIDER

Stress and fear frequently accompany pain, but when these emotional experiences significantly or consistently interfere with daily life, it is probably time to check in with an expert. For some children, prolonged stress or fear-based avoidance can evolve into an anxiety or depressive disorder, which can only make recovering from pain more difficult. If you feel concerned about a child's persistent stress, significant fear or avoidance of many situations, or increasing difficulty getting through the day, seek guidance from a behavioral health provider who has experience with helping children to manage pain and stress. (For detailed information on how to find and work successfully with such a professional, see Chapter 6.)

4

Managing Negativity, Frustration, and Doubt

Many children with pain and medical stress will say "This will never end," or "This is ruining my life." Even children who don't openly express these thoughts may harbor these fears or concerns. Parents, too, when they're in the thick of their child's medical evaluation and treatment, may feel this despair and aggravation. Perhaps you've thought, "It's so unfair that my child has to suffer," or "My child's doctors don't understand how horrible this is."

Negativity, frustration, and doubt are normal responses to any challenging situation and are common and understandable for families struggling with chronic pain. Yet parents may feel that a child's negative feelings are an inevitable result of the pain and overlook the possibility that negative feelings may additionally be a perpetuating factor in a chronic pain cycle.

While most parents can identify that their child has negativity, frustration, and doubt, it's less common for parents to understand that these feelings directly relate to their child's experience of pain. Additionally, these feelings may influence pain behaviors such as staying home from school, isolating from friends, and opting out of normal daily activities. As an early step in pain management, then, it is very important to help parents and children learn to modify negative feelings.

You might be thinking that this is a simple problem to fix: you could just change your feelings by telling yourself, "Okay, I won't get upset about this anymore." But research demonstrates that we can't just turn off these emotions by telling ourselves we won't *feel* this way. Instead, we have to change what we are *thinking* and *doing* to really change how we feel.

For example, imagine you're in the supermarket and in a rush to get home to your child who is counting the minutes until you return. Someone cuts in front of you in line. You are really annoyed. You're so annoyed that you'd like to give that rude person a piece of your mind. Now tell yourself to just stop being angry. Just stop. Right now.

You probably couldn't do it. Nor can most people.

In order to let go of the anger, you first have to learn how to change your *thinking*. For example, what if you thought to yourself: "She's probably in more of a rush than I am." Or maybe you could reason, "I was distracted looking at the magazines in line, so she probably didn't realize I was also waiting to check out." Immediately the anger and annoyance begin to subside and you feel calmer.

Now imagine that you went a step further and actively changed your behavior in this situation. Instead of continuing to focus on the problem or making a scene, what if you looked for another checkout line with a shorter wait and moved over? That *behavior* would decrease your anger and annoyance as well.

If you both modify your thinking and change your behavior, you're much more likely to feel better emotionally about the situation. Then you can move forward with your day and not hold on to feelings of anger and frustration. This is what you need to teach yourself and your own child to do in regard to his or her pain.

Because negative thoughts, frustrations, and doubts as they relate to pain and illness frequently vary by age, I've divided this section into the following three age groups; early childhood (4–7 years), middle-childhood (8–12 years), and adolescence (13–18 years). If your child's age falls near a transition point, you will probably want to read both of the sections that may apply.

Early Childhood: Ages 4–7

Preschool and early school-age children are often preoccupied with issues of safety. For most children ages four to seven, things that are perceived as threatening, such as pain, can induce negativity, frustration, and doubt and can lead to acting out or avoidance behaviors. Children at this stage of development really don't understand how the body works, and they aren't really able to learn about it in any sort of complicated way, so they may make up things to fill in the gaps. Often they end up with either a partially correct understanding or one that is pretty far off base. In general, children at this age try to fit what they don't know into a framework that is comfortable or familiar.

Young children may base their thinking about medical tests and procedures on something that is familiar, such as their experience with an elderly relative who was ill and ultimately died, or a movie they saw in which a single bad pain indicated a serious health issue. Or some children may feel their pain is a punishment for something bad they have done. Because children this age can't fully understand what is going on from a medical perspective, pain, illness, medical tests, and doctor visits can seem very scary, unpredictable, or even cruel. Seeing parents' negativity, frustration, and doubt only fuels their belief that something really bad is happening.

Consider Aiden, one of my young patients with recurrent migraine headaches. Aiden was a sweet, bright, sensitive, and very verbal child who had just started first grade when his headache pain ramped up. Before his headaches started, he had adored school. He was well liked by his classmates and teachers and was doing very well academically. So it really took his parents by surprise when he started saying, "I don't want to go school." They thought, understandably, that his pain was really interfering with his ability to enjoy school.

Early in our work together, however, we discovered that Aiden thought his headaches were contagious. He had learned that germs could be spread between classmates and worried that others in his class, including his teacher, would catch his headaches, too. He thought it was safer for everyone if he just stayed home. Through our work together Aiden learned to change how he *thought* about the situation (in particular, he learned that unlike a virus, a migraine headache can't be "caught"), which in turn changed what he *did* about the situation. He was able to attend school without the fear of infecting his classmates. Making these changes made him *feel* much more relaxed, which in turn helped to reduce the overall frequency and severity of his headaches.

I've learned over the years that it's easy to miss the misunderstandings or false associations that may be contributing to a young child's negativity, frustration, and doubt. Children don't know they're making connections that aren't really logical (because they seem quite logical to them), and these gaps of misinformation often fly under the radar. Additionally, sometimes an adult's first try at an explanation doesn't help. Negative thoughts, frustrations, or fears that have been in place for a long time can be tricky to unravel.

Middle Childhood: Ages 8–12

Children in middle childhood are just beginning to understand their bodies and how they work, but like younger children, they can often be confused regarding pain and illness and this can be a significant source of negativity, frustration, and doubt. While children at this age are becoming slightly more independent, they still rely heavily on parents and other adults in their world to keep them safe and teach them how to manage new situations.

For children in this age group, there is often a linear connection between hurt and harm: if it hurts, it must be harmful. This is a straightforward way of thinking about pain, but it doesn't always hold true in the world of chronic pain, where children with pain often don't have broken bones, torn ligaments, or a degenerative disease to explain their symptoms. This linear mindset also means that children at this stage of development often misinterpret body signs and symptoms. For example, I recently worked with a sweet eight-year-old girl named Rose who had chronic abdominal pain. When I met Rose she was at the end of a yearlong series of medical evaluations that included too many blood tests, scopes, ultrasounds, and medications to count. She was unhappy and was grasping to make sense of her symptoms and her very difficult year.

When I first spoke with Rose, I asked her what she thought was causing her pain. She said there was something wrong with her belly. I asked her to draw what she thought was wrong and she drew a self-portrait that included an enormous dark blob that enveloped her entire midsection. She said it felt like there was a rock in her belly, and she figured that eventually a test would reveal this "rock" and then doctors could remove it. She was frustrated that her doctors hadn't found what was wrong yet and said she felt really sad that no one knew what to do about the pain in her belly. I acknowledged her concern by sharing that I would also feel sad and frustrated if I thought I had a big rock in my belly that no one would remove.

With targeted education we were able to get Rose on board with the idea that tiny little nerves misbehaving in her belly were the cause of her pain, not a big rock. We then worked to break her association between hurt and harm by explaining that her brain may be sending pain signals, but this did not mean she needs surgery or that she will get worse. She was then able to modify her negative thoughts and feel more hopeful that this problem could be managed.

Adolescence: Ages 13–18

Many parents recognize and expect that a modicum of increased negativity, frustration, and doubt is an inherent part of adolescent development. While this is true, normal development at this time is not characterized by perpetual negativity, irritability, sadness, or self-doubt. Two of the major goals in adolescence are the development of personal autonomy and the creation of a "true" self that can navigate family, peer, and cultural expectations with confidence and a sense of well-being. When chronic pain emerges in adolescence it can derail these important developmental goals and this is often an underlying source of negativity, frustration, and doubt.

From a neurobiological perspective, adolescent brain development continues to about age twenty-four. Throughout this period, adolescents are gaining the capacity for good judgment, planning, and sound decision making, but they still need significant support from their parents. That is, although adolescents can understand most things about their bodies and know generally how to care for themselves, they often still require monitoring. This can be a very tricky task for parents, since adolescents may strongly resent parents' "nagging" about medicine or medical tests or about prescribed interventions such as physical therapy. They may feel their parents are over-involved in their lives and resent that they do not have as much freedom as their peers. Adolescents may think "I don't want to be different from my friends," or "This isn't fair," which may lead them to feel sad, isolated, or even hopeless. These feelings, in turn, often lead them to do . . . nothing. It's not logical, but indeed sometimes adolescents would rather do nothing than adhere to a promising pain-management plan. This negativity and inaction may be linked in part to a learned helplessness response. Repeated exposures to pain in the absence of feeling any sense of control over the pain can lead adolescents to feel that nothing will help. These feelings of futility and negativity make it difficult to muster the energy or interest needed to try new pain management strategies. When a learned helplessness response is in place, parents are charged with the task of helping their child to understand that it is possible to gain increased control over the management of pain.

Relatedly, some adolescents with pain may experience negative feelings associated with new or impending challenges. Consider that when children have pain they appear vulnerable, fragile, unstable, and weak. Even when they work hard to present a sturdier self to peers, teachers, and coaches, parents often see this less robust image of their adolescent. This presentation may unconsciously serve a purpose for adolescents. In some cases when adolescents are not quite ready to take on the developmental challenges of adolescence, or to tackle the normal transitions ahead (such as entering high school or preparing for college), their vulnerable presentation may be a signal that cues additional parent support and involvement in their day-to-day lives. This may at some level feel sweet and loving, but an adolescent who soaks up more parent involvement when he or she should be making some independent waves in the world is unfortunately not making progress toward important developmental goals and may continue to experience feelings of negativity, frustration, and doubt. When parents allow the adolescent to be stuck in this dependent state, they communicate a concern that the pain will not improve and a doubt that life will ever get back to normal, which further complicates recovery.

In general, it is enormously helpful to acknowledge your child's negative thoughts, frustrations, and doubts. But it's equally as important to teach and model for your child how to recognize and modify these feelings. This is a critical part of learning to manage a chronic pain experience.

◆

How to Help

1. USE THE REFLECTIVE LISTENING TECHNIQUE

Reflective listening is a communication strategy that works for children of any age. It's extremely effective for addressing feelings of negativity, frustration, and doubt, and a proven parent-based strategy for fostering and maintaining a strong emotional connection to your child. The process of reflective listening also helps a child to express his or her negative feelings and opens the door for problem-solving solutions. Don't give up if it doesn't work the first time you try it; with consistency most parents find this to be a keystone strategy. Here are the basic steps:

Listen. Your child's negative thoughts are probably so common and possibly so aligned with your own thinking that you may be missing them. Tune in to comments such as "This will never end," "Why me?," "No one understands this problem," "I can't do anything," or "My life is ruined." When you hear these comments, stop what you are doing and be sure to look your child in the eye so she knows that you are sincere and truly listening.

Reflect. Acknowledge these negative thoughts and comments by saying things like "I hear you," "It sounds like today is a very difficult day," "This feels very unfair to you." Give your child your full attention for a few moments. It's okay to share your child's frustration. Having chronic pain is frustrating and unfair. If your child stomps her foot and says, "This is so unfair," you can reflect this thought by joining with your child's frustration and agreeing, "Yes, this *is* unfair!" It's important for children to know that their parents are on their team and that their emotions, whatever they are, are valid. Once you have acknowledged these difficult feelings, however, it's critical that you take the next step of helping your child to manage this negativity and stay focused on the problem-solving strategies. It's perfectly normal for your child to vent about his or her situation, but ruminating, or frequently thinking about the negative aspects of the situation, is not productive.

Label, then validate, your child's feelings. Take a guess at how your child may be feeling by saying things like, "It sounds like you are really sad today," "I hear how angry you are feeling," "You seem so worried this afternoon." This is a really important step and will help you to uncover your child's feelings of negativity, frustration, and doubt. Interestingly, if you guess your child's feelings incorrectly, your child will almost certainly correct you by saying things like, "I'm not worried, I'm just mad at everyone," or "I'm not sad, I'm just feeling that this sucks." Once parents have labeled or identified negative feelings, they then need to *validate* their child's emotion. When parents say, "Don't feel so sad," or "You don't need to worry," children may feel that their parents don't understand their struggles. Even more importantly, trying to fix a child's feelings by telling him or her *not* to feel that way does not work. Remember that we have to change *thinking* and *behavior* to address negative feelings. Conversely, when parents validate a child's feelings by saying things like "Yes, I understand why you would feel that way today," or "Thank you for sharing with me how hard this is," children feel well understood and, importantly, are more open to problem-solving approaches.

Suggest an alternate way to think about the situation. After acknowledging your child's negative thoughts and emotions (with an "I hear you," "It sounds like you're really upset today," or another phrase), help your child to understand that changing how we think actually changes how we feel by brainstorming other ways to think about the situation. For example, if your child says "I can't do anything," help to move your child toward the more realistic thought "There are some things I can't do right now because I have pain and that is frustrating, but there are many things that I can do." Or if your child says "I can't take this anymore," you can acknowledge this negative thought (for example, "You sound really overwhelmed today"), then help to move him toward the thought that "I am really uncomfortable at the moment, but I know this will pass."

Encourage problem-solving. When children feel that their negative feelings are validated, they are primed to start thinking about how to address problems. Parents can encourage kids to take the lead with this by saying things like, "What do you think will help today?" or "What are you planning to do to get through this tough patch?" Notice that the questions are framed to encourage a child to take the next step. Avoid the pitfall of trying to jump in to solve your child's difficulty right away.

2. ADDRESS FALSE ASSOCIATIONS

Take the time to explain that, as strange as it may seem, pain doesn't always mean that something is wrong with the body, and even if your child knows someone with a similar pain, that person may have a very different problem. Read developmentally appropriate books about the body to help explain how things really work and make sure that your child has good resources at hand. Keep in mind that many children will try to look things up on the Internet before asking parents or doctors for information, and there is a lot of unreliable and sometimes very scary information available online. It can be helpful for parents and children to research together on the Internet so parents can ensure that their children are getting information from trusted websites such as those from major medical centers. (See Appendix 1 for suggestions.)

3. USE "THOUGHT STOPPING" COMBINED WITH DISTRACTION

Sit down with your child and make a list of her five most common negative thoughts. Then draw or imagine (in great detail) a big red stop sign. Your child needs to think of that stop sign every time one of those negative thoughts comes up. You can make a game out of it. Every time your child shares one of the negative thoughts from the list, say "Stop!" then help your child to get busy with a favorite activity. It may seem silly at first, but research has shown that the less time we spend thinking negative thoughts, the better we feel.

4. MODIFY YOUR CHILD'S "PAIN STORY"

A pain story is the story that parents and kids tell about all the testing, doctor appointments, medications, and challenges that they've faced. Pain stories tend to highlight feelings of desperation, negativity, futility, frustration, and doubt. While these stories may be accurate representations of a family's struggle to manage chronic pain, the more that children and parents tell this story, the more they come to adopt these feelings and to believe that their situation is very dire. A pain story that includes feelings of futility, anxiety, and doubt can perpetuate negativity and pain. Modify your child's pain story to downplay difficulties and to promote more positive thoughts. Work toward making your child the hero of the story, not the victim. Even if you don't feel positive about the situation, work toward framing the story in a more positive way. For example, you could say, "This situation has been challenging, but we're getting back on track," or "Yes, we've seen a lot of doctors, but I'm learning this can be managed." You will be very surprised to see how much better this modified story will make both you and your child feel. If you really need to communicate your frustration or negative thoughts to others, do not let your child overhear the conversation. Even young children hear and internalize much more than you may realize.

You should also help your child rewrite the story that he can tell others. Suggest appropriate words and phrases to say if your child needs this help. Be sure to create both a short and long version of the story so your child can use it in a variety of situations. (See Chapter 18.)

5. FAKE IT

Children of all ages rely heavily on their parents for cues about how to respond in various situations. Even if you are feeling frustrated, sad, or in despair, and feel like your negative thoughts will never go away, you want to communicate that negative feelings are only temporary. Work toward keeping a calm and confident attitude. As a bonus, you will be pleasantly surprised to find that "faking it" can help you feel better. In other words, by acting like things are getting back on track, your thinking will actually change, and you will start to feel more positive and less frustrated.

6. DON'T APOLOGIZE FOR YOUR CHILD'S PAIN

Parents often say "I'm sorry" when their child reports pain or negative thoughts. Your child's pain is not your fault and you should not take the blame. By apologizing you imply that you should do something to make the situation better. As you make your way through this book you will learn how your child can start to own this difficulty and feel empowered in the process. Just acknowledge negative thoughts or feelings and then move on without apologizing.

7. TRY NOT TO OVER-IDENTIFY WITH YOUR CHILD

It's important to keep your experiences separate from those of your child. If you often say things like "We are not having a good day today," you may be over-identifying with your child. Parents typically make "we" statements in an effort to unite with their child, and many parents really do feel their child's pain so deeply that when their child is having a bad day, the parent truly is having a bad day too. Even so, in the counterintuitive world of pain management, using "we" statements tends to make the problem worse. Children and adolescents commonly report that they feel guilty for having chronic pain. They fully recognize the strain this places on the family and on the parents in particular. They are aware when parents must miss work or activities to take them to the doctor, they quickly pick up on the financial burden associated with chronic pain, and they recognize the stress it places on parents' lives. So when parents imply that their child's pain has also directly led to their having pain or a bad day, they increase their child's feelings of negativity and frustration. In addition, the use of "we" statements can unintentionally suggest to children that parents should bear more responsibility for improving the pain, when in fact we want children to feel empowered to do more in this situation. Parents should instead help their child to express his or her individual feelings with the use of the reflective listening technique, and acknowledge that there may be days that are better and days that are worse.

8. DON'T REACT EMOTIONALLY TO YOUR CHILD'S EMOTION

Children will not share their feelings openly if parents become upset or spiral into a state of anxiety when they express their negative feelings, frustrations, or doubt. Maintaining open communication and helping your child with negativity mean that parents must find a way to maintain a calm and collected attitude when their child expresses these negative feelings. Additionally, parents should resist the urge to jump into action to try to fix negative emotions or the stressors that caused them. Instead, parents are encouraged to respond calmly in a way that conveys to their child that they can tolerate and accept their child's negative feelings, and are available to support their child in making adaptive changes.

9. MODEL HOW TO REDUCE NEGATIVITY

One of the best things that parents can do is talk about how they manage negative thoughts on a bad day. The more parents describe out loud how they cope with life's frustrations, disappointments, and curveballs by using more positive thinking and actions, the more their children will adopt these strategies, too.

5

Redefining Comfort

At its core, this is a book about comfort. Specifically, it's about how to help generate feelings of comfort for your child no matter what type of pain or pain-related stress your child is experiencing. The challenge is that creating comfort for a child with pain requires parents to think way outside the "rest on the couch with hot cocoa until you feel better" box. We need to support and enable a child's core of comfort, the kind of comfort that is associated with a positive outlook, a sense of resilience, and feelings of self-efficacy. Kids who have these core elements of comfort are more likely to be able to effectively manage pain at home, in school, and with friends. They also tend to have lives that are less disrupted by pain or illness.

Snuggling on the couch, sleeping late, watching TV, and playing video games are all fun and well-established sources of comfort for most children and adolescents, but for those in pain, these remedies usually lose their effectiveness over time and so are useful only as a quick fix. In other words, kids who lie on the couch for days or weeks at a time may look relaxed playing their games or watching TV. But after working with these kids in therapy for many years I have come to understand that in truth they rack up an enormous amount of pain-related stress just sitting on the couch. Children are well aware that every day they spend on the couch means that they are falling further behind in school while missing out on sport practices, family activities, and fun with friends. They may also notice, often with guilt, that their family members have had to change their schedules and commitments to accommodate their pain. I think that most kids recognize at some level, too, that resting too much makes them feel worse. They just don't know another way.

In order to help your child to develop more comfort, it's helpful to first think about how you would define comfort for your child. Keep in mind that being comfortable is not just about being without pain. If your child hates to be cold, then part of comfort might include being dressed warmly on a cold day or being wrapped in a toasty blanket. If your child enjoys Grandma's famous spaghetti and meatballs, then part of comfort might include having a full belly after this delicious meal. If your child loves the outdoors, then part of comfort might include taking a hike through the woods. If your child loves school, then part of comfort might include getting a good grade on a tough test. Perhaps comfort is all of those things for your child. Or perhaps none of those is really part of comfort for your child. When it comes down to it, defining comfort is a very individual exercise. What's comfortable for one person may not be comfortable for another. Many parents may also notice that their child's preferred comfort strategy changes depending on the setting. For example, an eight-year-old child may crawl into a parent's lap for comfort at a doctor's appointment, but would not seek a parent's lap for comfort at a school event where her peers might notice.

When I discuss the broader context of comfort with parents in my clinical practice, I ask parents to think about their child's comfort in several settings such as at home, in school, and with peers. In this way we can uncover how a child finds comfort in various settings. Knowing this helps when creating a plan to increase comfort in places where it is lacking. Children almost universally report that the easiest place to attain comfort is at home. It feels safe and secure, and while at home, kids don't have to worry much about their response to pain because they can generally control their environment to manage their symptoms: they can turn off the lights, use the computer or TV as a distraction, take medications, use heating pads, stretch out on a bed, ask Mom or Dad for support, and so on. When I work with parents and children around building home-based comforts, my efforts are usually focused on trying to get families to shake up their routines. I try to move kids away from more passive and dependent aspects of comfort (resting on the couch watching TV, snuggling with a parent) to more active and independent skills that produce comfort (taking a short walk, engaging in relaxation skills). The reason for this shift is that when kids come to think of home as the only place where they can obtain comfort, they often start to struggle in their efforts to obtain comfort elsewhere. Conversely, when kids feel that many of the effective strategies they use at home (such as breathing techniques, or taking a break to walk or stretch) can be used while away from home—at a friend's house, say, or a school event— they will feel more confident about leaving the cocoon of the house and restoring a more normal balance to their daily routine.

As a general rule, we want children to have the confidence that they can find a kind of comfort that suits them at any particular time and in any setting. This confidence is often termed "self-efficacy" and is part of what helps children of all ages to be resilient in the management of chronic pain.

Comfort and Resilience

Think of resilience as your child's ability to "bounce." Some kids are born bouncy. They seem to move through the world without much difficulty. Every time they encounter a bump in the road, they just bounce right over it with hardly a care. Other kids seem to have far less bounce: when they hit a similar bump in the road, they get stuck. We all want to have bouncy kids. But temperament, genes, injury, illness, stress, and loads of other factors can conspire to take the bounce right out of them. Your child may have been a bouncy kid until pain or illness got in the way. Or you may have a child who never really bounced very well and pain or illness has only made the problem worse. The good news is that bounciness as it relates to pain, pain-related stress, and disability can be taught. The goal is to help children to realize that they can learn to bounce, even in the context of pain.

Research shows that resilience changes the relationship between pain and overall adaptation. People with chronic pain who are resilient are more upbeat, are better able to participate in daily activities, and generally feel more successful than people who are not resilient. For people with pain, the key to resilience is rooted in feelings of self-efficacy. When we talk about pain-related self-efficacy we want to know specifically: How confident does your child feel about managing pain at school, or around friends at a party?; How confident does your child feel that he or she can be active even when experiencing some pain? Many children with chronic or recurrent pain have very low confidence on these fronts.

In research I've conducted, parents and children seem to agree when it comes to a child's level of self-efficacy in managing his or her pain. When kids have low pain-related self-efficacy, parents also rate them as having low self-efficacy. When kids have confidence in their ability to manage pain, parents see that too. Changes in pain-related self-efficacy don't occur overnight, but they can happen faster than you might think. When parents have confidence that their children have the skills and supports they need to effectively manage their own pain, and see their child as someone who is capable of solving a pain-related difficulty on his or her own, children start to see themselves that way too. But parents may have to show their children through their beliefs and behaviors that they know their kids can bounce before kids can see themselves as bouncy, too.

To help foster a child's sense of self-efficacy and his or her belief that pain can be managed, parents should:

1. Remember that long-term comfort does not come from resting at home or withdrawing from situations, places, or people.

2. Redefine comfort as a feeling of well-being that comes from very personalized, individualized preferences and that stems, in part, from feelings of self-efficacy in valued activities like school, sports, and hobbies.
3. Think about comfort as something that ideally can happen at home, in school, and with friends. Work toward increasing your child's sense of self-efficacy in those situations and places where he or she is not fully engaged, lacks confidence, or experiences stress or discomfort.
4. Adopt a parent-goes-first attitude about your child's pain-related self-efficacy. Remember that when you believe your child has, or can have again, resilience or "bounce," your child will be more likely to start to think of herself in that way too.

◆

How to Help

1. CONSTRUCT A COMFORT GUIDE

Together with your child, think about a time when things were going well and your child experienced comfort from many sources. What was going on in your child's life at that time? What brought comfort to your child? Make a list of the activities that gave your child a sense of comfort and happiness. Perhaps your list will include some of the following activities:

> Learning a new song on the piano
> Volunteering at a soup kitchen
> Helping a sibling with homework
> Playing beach Frisbee
> Snuggling with a pet
> Learning to bake or cook
> Reading a great book
> Taking a hot bath
> Listening to music

Playing in the yard
Scoring a goal in a soccer game
Participating in student government
Marching in the school band
A good night's sleep
Earning a good grade on a test
Going on a family vacation
Helping a neighbor
Winning a baseball game
Drawing or painting
Planning a sleepover
Playing a video game
Going to a movie
Being surrounded by close friends
A day with nothing scheduled
A delicious meal
Cooking dinner for the family
Winning a competition
Performing in a play
Feeling accomplished
Making people laugh
Going for a hike
Cheering on a favorite sports team
Learning a new skill
Taking good care of a pet
Snuggling with a favorite toy or blanket
Getting together with cousins or relatives

Now take a look at the experiences you noted. Some of these activities may be possible to do now, and some may be out of reach due to your child's pain. Talk about this with your child. With your child, pick a few items that could be part of a current comfort-boosting routine, and brainstorm together about some that could be part of a future plan (you can even rank the activities from easiest to hardest, to help with your planning). Add more comfort-boosting activities to your list as you're talking. Then shake up your current routines by adding in a dose of these comfort-boosting activities and talking about your child's experience afterward (but don't ask about his pain!). Remember to give plenty of encouragement and support, and to acknowledge your child's own efforts to take this important step toward greater independence and self-efficacy.

2. REMEMBER TOGETHER A "BOUNCY" TIME

Was there a difficulty with a mean child at school that your child navigated on his or her own? Has your child solved conflicts with a sibling without you stepping in to help? Has your child made new friends after moving to a new neighborhood or switching schools? Has your child been faced with a previous illness, injury, or life adversity and figured out a plan for managing the problem? Whether the bounce is big or small doesn't matter. To start your conversation, you need just one example of how your child rose to the occasion and showed some good problem-solving skills. Then talk about the idea of "bounce" with your child, describing pain, illness, or medical stress as simply another bump in the road.

You can work together to think of ways to bounce, but be sure to let your child lead the way. Sometimes children will come up with solutions that will surprise you. Whatever they suggest, validate their suggestions with comments such as "I can see how that could help."

3. REMEMBER THAT COMFORT AND PAIN CAN COEXIST

By more broadly defining comfort, kids will discover that they can more easily find ways to engage and succeed in multiple activities—and so find social, emotional, or sensorial comfort—perhaps even while feeling pain. This discovery is often a huge revelation for kids and hopefully for parents too. Of course we want children's pain and pain-related stress to disappear. For some that will most certainly happen and for others there may be some elements of pain that recur or persist.

Whatever course your child's pain may take, he or she needs to know that finding effective ways to access comfort from various sources along the way will only help with the pain and the negative feelings that can accompany pain symptoms.

4. TAKE A STEP BACK

Parents often get stuck believing that they need to continue to provide comfort for their child until their child steps up to the plate. But once you've worked with your child to more broadly define comfort and come up with some specific activities or aspects of comfort that your child can access in various settings, it's time to start relinquishing your role as a daily back-rubber or pillow fluffer. Taking a step back is an essential kind of support. In fact, letting your child take the lead in identifying and re-engaging with favorite forms of comfort can help to build a sense of self-efficacy, which is an essential step in bolstering resilience and fostering your child's overall recovery.

Part II

Get Ready: Selecting Evidence-Based Treatments

If you search on the Internet for "child pain management" you will receive almost 30 million hits. Yes, 30 *million*. And this number is growing every day. There are many resources and providers who offer treatments for children with pain. Not surprisingly, however, a significant number of these resources are unlikely to be effective, and a few may even be harmful to children. For this reason, I always caution my patients and their parents to be wary consumers when investigating pain-management resources and treatments.

The reality is that only a few treatments are "evidence-based," which means that they are supported by strong, peer-reviewed research. These are the gold-standard treatments and they should be the cornerstones of your child's pain treatment plan. Other treatments that offer preliminary or growing evidence supporting their use in children with pain may bolster or enhance recovery and coping efforts, but still should be used with caution. The pros and cons of these interventions should be considered carefully before initiating treatment.

This section of the book is devoted to helping parents wade through the sea of treatment options. While the science is always evolving, the next few chapters are intended to shed light on the current state of our knowledge in pediatric pain management: which interventions are known to be helpful, which interventions might be worthwhile, and those interventions that should in most cases be avoided.

One topic that comes up quickly in discussions about pain treatments is the use of complementary and alternative medicine treatments. The management of pain and medical stress is often a very individual experience, and different children respond differently to various interventions. It's important to keep an open mind, then, and to consider that complementary and alternative medicine treatments may offer significant comfort and support, especially when combined with more conventional approaches to pain management.

In most comprehensive pain services, three branches of intervention form the trifecta of rehabilitation for chronic pain: behavioral medicine interventions, physical or occupational therapy, and targeted pain-management medications. These interventions receive the highest recommendations because they are evidence-based with solid research to support their effectiveness. These are the cornerstones of a good multidisciplinary plan, and they may be administered in a packaged format, as is the case in many pediatric rehabilitation centers, or pieced together in a comprehensive outpatient treatment plan. In both instances these interventions seem to have a whole that is greater than the sum of their parts. In other words, while they all demonstrate independent effectiveness, it seems that when they are administered together they have an even greater benefit. For this reason, when these interventions are prescribed, we strongly suggest that parents initiate all three interventions at the same time. Trying one intervention and then moving to the next may not be as effective and can slow progress.

Behavioral medicine, structured physical activity, and medications are such important interventions that each one is detailed in its own chapter. Behavioral medicine interventions, including cognitive behavioral therapy, mindfulness, biofeedback, and self-hypnosis, are detailed in Chapter 6; physical and occupational therapy are detailed in Chapter 7; and medications and supplements for chronic pain are reviewed in Chapter 8. Parents need to have the facts about how and why these interventions work so they can be educated consumers for their children.

Beyond behavioral medicine, structured physical activity, and medications, there are many other interventions that may offer additional benefit. Chapter 9 describes many of the most popular strategies in detail and explains why they are, or are not, commonly recommended for children with pain.

Without a doubt, chronic pain management requires a team approach, as well as a combination of therapies. When a person is struggling with chronic pain I often say that they are like a car with four flat tires. We need to fill all of the tires in order to get going again. Medication might fill one tire, but multiple interventions—including behavioral medicine, physical therapy, and others—are most likely needed to help the car get back on its way. If you are new to the idea of a multidisciplinary therapeutic approach, it will be wise to consult with your child's primary care doctor or pain-management specialist about additional interventions that may be best for your child. If you and your child are already using this approach, now is a good time to review the selection of interventions that are in place and think about where you may be able to modify your child's plan to maximize success.

6

Behavioral Medicine

I have a love-hate relationship with the term "behavioral medicine." It emerged in the 1970s at a conference at Yale University where some thoughtful, passionate physicians argued that pain and illness are best conceptualized in a biopsychosocial framework. In other words, we can't view a person's pain or illness (the biological part) without also considering the psychological and social aspects of that person's world. This health model quickly rose to prominence and still today guides our collective understanding of pain, illness, and coping. The psychologically based therapies that target pain and pain-related difficulties—that is, the behavioral component of behavioral medicine—have come to play a leading role in pain management overall.

But since this term was first used, "behavioral medicine" has also come to refer, imprecisely, to many different types of psychological therapy. It seems like "behavioral medicine" is now often the softer, gentler, or more popular way to refer to various psychological interventions. But behavioral medicine is not just any psychological therapy, and this mixup in definitions has caused a lot of frustration for families who seek targeted services.

The term "behavioral medicine," when used correctly, refers to a particular set of psychological strategies that addresses a wide range of health-related issues. When children with chronic pain or illness use these tried-and-true interventions, they usually are able to cope, do more of their usual activities, feel like their lives are getting back on track, and may also have less pain. But with alternative meanings for "behavioral medicine" flying around, parents may think they are getting a targeted behavioral medicine intervention for their child when in fact they are receiving something else entirely. We can't undo what's been done to this term. But when parents learn what behavioral medicine interventions are, and how they target pain, they can make informed decisions about the specific types of psychologically based interventions that are available to them.

This chapter reviews the gold-standard behavioral medicine strategies for managing pain: cognitive-behavioral therapy, self-hypnosis, biofeedback, and mindfulness. These strategies are well-tested and proven to help children with chronic pain get back on track.

Remember that initiating services for behavioral medicine does not imply that pain is a psychological problem. Yet because chronic pain is commonly associated with stressors such as sleep disruptions, school-based challenges, and loss of social connections, it is linked to a higher risk for psychological difficulties such as anxiety and depression. Research shows that kids with chronic pain have three times the risk of having a psychological disorder as compared to the general pediatric population. This means that approximately 20 to 35 percent of children with chronic pain will also meet diagnostic criteria for a psychological disorder. Research also suggests that having both chronic pain and a psychological disorder leads to worse disability. Fortunately, behavioral medicine interventions can simultaneously target pain, pain-related stress, and many types of psychological disorders.

Cognitive-Behavioral Therapy

Cognitive-behavioral therapy (CBT) is the most commonly researched and most proven psychological treatment for the management of pediatric pain. CBT is a brief, goal-oriented psychotherapy treatment that takes a hands-on, practical approach to problem-solving. It is based on the idea that thoughts, feelings, and behaviors are all connected. Because people can learn to control their thoughts, it is possible to change feelings and behaviors even when a problem, such as chronic pain, does not immediately go away. Within a CBT practice for pediatric pain, children are taught *thought-based strategies* to identify and restructure unhelpful thoughts related to pain. Children are also taught *behavioral strategies* to relieve discomfort and improve functioning.

For example, a child with a chronic pain condition such as complex regional pain syndrome in her foot would be taught that she would not cause harm to herself by using that foot. Her treatment would then address the negative or fearful thoughts (such as "it's going to hurt too much to walk") that produce both physiologic changes (for example, racing heart, shortness of breath, increased discomfort) and behavioral changes (perhaps a withdrawal from activity). The child would be taught to alter the thoughts, saying to herself something like "Walking may be temporarily uncomfortable, but it will help me get back to my activities and I can use my coping skills to get through it." The goal is to reduce the uncomfortable physical reactions to the idea of trying something challenging and instead promote more adaptive responses that build the child's sense of confidence and self-efficacy. CBT can also directly address unhelpful behavioral responses to pain, such as avoidance of activities like attending school, with the use of strategies such as "graded exposure" (in this case, slowly increasing the child's time at school over days and weeks) and reinforcement for positive changes in behaviors. (This approach is detailed in Chapter 16.)

Relaxation strategies are almost always a part of the CBT approach to chronic pain. Relaxation skills can ease pain and reduce physiological stress. These strategies produce real and meaningful changes in heart rate, body temperature, breathing, oxygen levels, blood pressure, hormone levels, and muscle tension. They can also improve the functioning of the immune system, digestive health, energy levels, and sleep. When children learn to use relaxation techniques on their own, too, they feel a greater sense of control over their bodies, which may both help counteract the feelings of helplessness that are frequently brought on by chronic pain and bolster feelings of self-efficacy. (Relaxation skills are detailed in Part 3.)

CBT is effective for pain management for several reasons. First, behaviorally based relaxation strategies such as diaphragmatic breathing, muscle relaxation, or guided imagery can decrease the sensation of pain. Second, CBT strategies can improve a child's ability to have a normally active day, even if the pain is not reduced. And third, pain and suffering are often linked to feelings of hopelessness, helplessness, frustration, fear, and anxiety. These feelings can exacerbate pain, interfere with medical care, increase disability, and contribute to ongoing symptoms of anxiety and depression. CBT can be very helpful for managing these negative thoughts and feelings. The overarching goals of CBT for pain include gaining a sense of control over pain, reducing stress and fear related to pain, improving daily function, increasing feelings of hopefulness and resourcefulness, and improving mood.

Variations on the CBT Theme

Over the past thirty years, several variations of CBT have emerged and gained in popularity. These newer variations of CBT, including contextual cognitive behavioral therapy (CCBT), dialectical behavioral therapy (DBT), and acceptance and commitment therapy (ACT), include most of the major tenets of CBT but generally place greater emphasis on the acceptance of pain or thoughts related to pain rather than on changing those thoughts. These theories also place more emphasis on staying focused in the present moment than traditional CBT does. ACT and CCBT for chronic pain management may be particularly helpful for kids who are feeling very stuck with their pain, who are making slower than expected progress with therapy, or who, due to underlying disease processes or other factors, are not likely to be able to ease their pain symptoms. It is important to note that the term "acceptance" does not imply giving in to pain or in any way resolving to continually experience pain. The goal of acceptance is to acknowledge that even if pain is present, it is possible to live a meaningful life. There is a limited but growing body of literature supporting the application of CCBT and ACT in kids with chronic pain. This literature offers promising evidence that the acceptance of pain may be an important way forward for children struggling with this difficult problem.

Other Behavioral Medicine Strategies

There are other research-proven skills that are helpful for managing chronic pain in children, whether or not they are incorporated into a CBT program. Beyond the use of CBT, then, parents should look for the following well-supported approaches:

MINDFULNESS

Mindfulness is the ability to remain focused in the present moment while ignoring everything else. For example, during mindfulness practice patients may be taught how to focus exclusively on a small object they are touching or a single bite of food in their mouth. When a child is fully engaged in thinking about her "in-the-moment" experience, she cannot also think about how long her pain will last, missed schoolwork, or how frustrated she feels. Many pediatric behavioral medicine specialists incorporate mindfulness-based skills into their CBT work with children who have chronic pain, and it is one of the primary skills used in ACT and DBT (for more information on mindfulness practice, see Chapter 13).

BIOFEEDBACK

Biofeedback simply means getting information from the body. During biofeedback, patients can see information about their physiology in real time on a computer screen or biofeedback device. For example, patients can see how quickly their heart is beating, how fast they are breathing, how much moisture their skin emits, how tense their muscles are, and their skin temperature, all of which are measures of our body's response to stress. Biofeedback can be a wonderful way for children to get concrete information about their physiological state and learn ways to make positive changes to this state. In particular, when children are experiencing severe pain, their nervous system is usually in a state of high arousal. Conversely, low arousal, or a state of relaxation, is generally incompatible with pain. Recent advances in biofeedback technology make the task of trying to relax particularly engaging for children and adolescents: an engaging video-game-like interface effectively distracts a child from thoughts of pain while at the same time heightening his or her attention to the goals of relaxation. While looking at the screen, kids can see exactly how their bodies respond when they engage in relaxation-based exercises (for more information on biofeedback, see Chapter 14).

SELF-HYPNOSIS

The idea of hypnosis is intriguing to some parents and very off-putting to others. But hypnosis has been around for hundreds of years and there is strong evidence that it provides relief to many people suffering from chronic pain. It has been cited in the literature as a treatment for pain since the 1840s, and while the techniques essentially have remained the same, our confidence in the strategy has grown. This is in part due to our increased understanding of the role our brain plays in processing pain. Impressively, functional imaging studies (fMRI) have shown that the brain responds differently to pain when a patient is in a state of hypnosis.

The hallmark feature of self-hypnosis is a state of altered consciousness. Anyone who has had a daydream has been in an altered state of consciousness, and so we all know that it's not actually scary and it is in no way associated with a loss of control. In fact, most people who use self-hypnosis actually report feeling a heightened sense of control.

Self-hypnosis simply involves teaching children to relax deeply and then shift their cognitive awareness away from pain, instead becoming fully absorbed in an imaginative experience. Once their conscious awareness has been shifted away from their pain, a provider can often make suggestions about physical sensations or movements that may be associated with symptom relief even after the hypnotic state has ended.

Younger children tend to be naturals at self-hypnosis: they already shift between real and imagined worlds effortlessly in their pretend play and can easily be taught to enter their imaginary worlds as a way to shift their attention away from pain. Older adolescents, by contrast, can find self-hypnosis to be challenging because they tend to be more guarded about shifting their attention away from present awareness. For this reason, it's sometimes easier for older adolescents to first learn some basic relaxation strategies before tackling the self-hypnosis techniques.

Parent and Family Interventions for Chronic Pain

No matter which psychologically based intervention your child is involved with, you, the parent, matter a great deal. Not surprisingly, then, while the development and testing of parent-focused treatments for pediatric pain are still evolving, there's enough evidence now to conclude that parent-focused interventions are associated with better outcomes for children with chronic pain. This makes perfect sense. When parents are distressed or don't know ideal strategies for supporting their kids, it's much harder for those kids to progress. Fortunately, it works the other way as well. When parents have a positive attitude and adhere to the strategies that are known to promote a child's recovery from pain and pain-related stress, kids do much better. New research suggests that psychological interventions that teach parents how to change their own responses to their child's pain and to develop pain- or illness-specific problem-solving skills have a lasting effect on a how a child manages pain. Though many of these parent-based strategies are described in this book, parents should advocate for the opportunity to learn more about these strategies if their child is working directly with a behavioral medicine provider.

Parents are also encouraged to take the time to assess thoughtfully their own level of distress. For example, if you recognize that you are anxious most of the time, feel overwhelmed when your child has pain, or have difficulty making decisions about your child's day-to-day activity, working with a behavioral medicine provider who uses a structured problem-solving therapy approach can be among one of the best things you can do for your child. (See Chapter 19 for more on parent self-care.)

◆

How to Help

1. LOCATE PROVIDERS IN THE U.S.

Finding referrals for behavioral medicine is not as tricky as some people think. In most cases, you don't even need a referral from a primary care provider to seek services; you just need to locate a good clinical therapist. The first step is to ask a pediatrician, primary care provider, or trusted friend for recommended providers. If you don't have luck there, you can call the number on the back of your insurance card for "behavioral medicine," "behavioral health," or "mental health support" to get a list of eligible providers who are covered by your insurance and who are located nearby. Often insurance carriers can pare down the list of providers by searching only for providers who work with children or adolescents, or who have a certain focus to their practices (such as chronic pain, CBT, or stress management). Parents can also search for a local provider by selecting the "find a CBT provider" link on the Association for Behavioral and Cognitive Therapists (ABCT) website: www.abct.org. Another idea is to call the American Psychological Association (APA) public education information line (1-800-964-2000), where operators will connect you to a referral system in your area.

2. CHECK FOR QUALIFICATIONS

Behavioral medicine providers have various qualifications; here's a quick lesson in who has what training. Providers with a Ph.D. in psychology have obtained five to seven years of doctoral training that focus on therapy and research. A child clinical or a clinical pediatric psychologist is an ideal candidate for working with a child who has chronic pain.

Providers with a Psy.D. have also obtained doctoral-level training in psychology. The Psy.D. is a newer doctorate-level designation for providers who have obtained four to five years of training in clinical therapy, with typically less research training than a traditional Ph.D. There are also child subspecialties within this field and parents should seek a Psy.D. provider with child or pediatric experience.

Clinicians who are called a "licensed independent clinical social worker" (LICSW) or "licensed mental health counselor" (LMHC), or have achieved a "masters in social work" (MSW), have received two years of graduate training in clinical therapy and/or resource management.

There may be other qualified providers available as well, but parents should be aware that unfortunately the field of mental health can include unlicensed providers without graduate-level training who may not be monitored by any professional organization, meaning that there is no way to ensure a standard of care or professional accountability.

3. SCREEN FOR SKILLS

If you are seeking behavioral medicine services for your child, be an informed consumer. Not all therapists have expertise in the behavioral medicine approaches reviewed in this chapter. Check out the providers' websites or simply call the providers to find out if they have experience treating chronic pain in children or adolescents. If so, ask if they use CBT, relaxation-based treatments, biofeedback, or mindfulness training in their work. If the answer is yes, you have likely found a qualified provider. If the providers you contact don't have experience with chronic pain, but do use CBT, relaxation-based treatments, biofeedback, self-hypnosis, and/or mindfulness training for other types of problems such as anxiety or depression, this could also be a good fit. Keep in mind that providers don't need to have all of the skills—for example, there are very few providers who do biofeedback with children—but the behavioral medicine strategies outlined in this chapter are the gold-standard therapeutic approaches for chronic pain. Talk therapy, or other more general supportive therapies, have not been proven through research to alleviate chronic pain problems. Be very choosy on the skills front.

4. PREPARE CHILDREN FOR TREATMENT

It is important for parents and children to have realistic expectations for CBT before the treatment begins. For example, the entire family must understand that participating in psychological pain-management strategies in no way implies that the pain itself is a psychological problem. It is also helpful to explain to children that behavioral medicine treatments for pain may not eliminate pain immediately or entirely, though it is common for kids with chronic pain to report that using these treatments makes the pain less noticeable and less disruptive to everyday life.

5. ASSESS FOR FIT

It's true that having a good "fit," or a strong personal connection, with a provider is important in a therapeutic relationship. But fit can be difficult to determine at first because it can take several sessions for parents and kids to feel like they have a good working relationship with a provider. I usually recommend that patients try at least four sessions before deciding whether they have a good fit with their provider. During the first "intake" session the provider usually collects a lot of information from parents and kids, but provides little intervention. The second and third sessions are often devoted to educating the parents and children about the therapy process, establishing a treatment plan, and building rapport. By the end of the fourth session, the first mostly therapeutic visit, both parties should know how they feel. Of course, there are exceptions to this rule; sometimes kids and parents know right away that it's a great fit, or that it just won't work. You can trust your instinct on this, but if you're on the fence give it some time before you decide.

6. FOLLOW THROUGH

The skills-based approach that guides CBT and other skills-based chronic pain interventions requires consistency. Your child will have homework most weeks and you should encourage your child to practice his or her skills regularly. Sometimes parents can practice with their child as a show of solidarity and support, and to demonstrate their commitment to the interventions. Parents should also be sure that their children keep scheduled weekly appointments, especially for the first eight to twelve sessions. After that, if your child has demonstrated good progress, it is sometimes possible to reduce the frequency of appointments to every other week.

7. STAY ENGAGED

Younger children (say, ages five to twelve) often require parental support during their treatment. Make sure you feel comfortable collaborating with your child's behavioral medicine provider and ask what you can do at home to reinforce your child's coping strategies and bolster their progress. Parents of younger children are also often included in parts of the therapeutic session so they can see their child's new skills in action and offer essential encouragement. Even though older adolescents will want and need a more private and autonomous relationship with their provider, and children of all ages need to develop a personal relationship with their provider as part of their healing process, parents should still keep up to speed about the general themes or skills being covered in their child's therapy.

8. PLAN AHEAD

Even after the full course of CBT has ended, it can be very useful to revisit the provider on an as-needed or "maintenance" basis, to help prevent relapses. Meeting every three to six months after a complete course of CBT treatment may help to reinforce newly learned skills and identify any new symptoms that have emerged before they become problematic. Additionally, a booster therapy session can help to maintain developmentally appropriate education and CBT skills to meet a child's changing needs.

9. SEEK PARENT- AND FAMILY-BASED SERVICES

Because parents are so critically important to their child's recovery, they should consider attending a parent group that can give them guidance about how best to facilitate their child's progress. Additionally, if parents themselves have persistent anxiety or mood-based challenges, now is the perfect time to seek professional help, for their child and for themselves. Family-based treatments or couples counseling can also be beneficial. See Chapter 19 for more information on these and other services.

7

Physical and Occupational Therapy

Over the past twenty years our understanding of the short- and long-term benefits of physical and occupational therapy for a wide range of pain-related difficulties has grown by leaps and bounds. If your child has felt limited physically by chronic pain, it can be useful to talk to your doctor about being evaluated for physical or occupational therapy. Physical and occupational therapists are experts in rehabilitation. They carefully evaluate your child's symptoms in the context of how she or he navigates daily activities at home and in school. They then establish a plan for rehabilitation based on your child's unique needs.

Physical Therapy

It turns out that physical therapy (PT) not only promotes healing at the level of the bone, muscle, and tendon, but also can modify the experience of pain within the brain and central nervous system. Moreover, physical therapists can often offer new insights into a child's persistent pain. A thorough PT evaluation can identify underlying causes of chronic pain as well as secondary factors that maintain pain cycles. For example, a physical therapist may find that a child with chronic back pain has flat feet, an irregular gait, or inward-turning knees. A child with chronic headache pain may be found to have poor cervical posture and muscle imbalances in the back and shoulders, which can place increased strain on the cervical spine and neck and so contribute to headaches.

Physical therapists are also experts at identifying factors that may exacerbate pain and in understanding how biomechanical differences can contribute to chronic pain cycles. For example, the child described earlier with back pain may receive advice on special shoes to wear to correct her flat feet, gait training to correct her improper gait, and recommendations for an adaptive device such as an orthotic to promote improved positioning of her ankles and knees. PT interventions also frequently address, with instruction and exercise, impairments such as decreased flexibility, pain arising from a damaged joint or muscle, areas of physical weakness, nerve hypersensitivity, poor balance, chronic fatigue, and general deconditioning. The goal is to teach patients to integrate recommended strategies into their daily lives, so they can maintain or build on the progress made in physical therapy.

Active Physical Therapy Interventions

Active PT interventions require that the child be an engaged participant in the intervention. During active PT, a physical therapist may teach a child how to do an exercise or activity, but the child must also actively do it.

GRADED PHYSICAL THERAPY AND ACTIVITY PACING

"Graded physical therapy" is by far the most common and proven intervention in physical therapy. This active technique has been demonstrated to reduce pain, improve physical function, and reduce the fear of pain in children and adolescents. A graded PT program is an individualized program. The first step is to determine a child's baseline function. Then a physical therapist works closely with the child and family to determine a challenging, but comfortable, rate at which to increase the child's activity level. The plan may include targeted exercises or stretches as well as activities of daily living (like walking to the bus stop, or taking the family dog for a walk). The plan is typically made in collaboration with the child and emphasizes the importance of the child actively participating in his or her own recovery.

AQUA THERAPY

Aqua therapy is sometimes suggested as the first step in a person's physical therapy because the water reduces the amount of pressure on the body, making movement more comfortable. When a person is immersed in water up to his waist, his weight is effectively reduced by 50 percent and when immersed up to his neck, his weight is reduced by 90 percent. This weight reduction creates buoyancy, which makes it significantly easier to move muscles and joints and gain the confidence needed to move a painful area. The water pressure can also help to decrease swelling and if the pool is heated, the warmth of the water can ease muscle tension or muscle spasms. Aqua therapy can also be used to improve a person's core strength and balance, as well as his or her overall physical condition. Once children can move easily in the water, they are typically advanced to a land-based intervention.

DESENSITIZATION

Desensitization is an intervention that is designed to make nerves less sensitive and it is especially useful for neuropathic pain conditions such as complex regional pain syndrome, where a painful area often becomes hypersensitive. In a desensitization protocol a PT will expose the painful area to various touches, temperature changes, or movements, starting with a neutral or only slightly uncomfortable touch and slowly working up to more normal activities. For example, in the case of a foot with neuropathic pain, a PT might start by lightly touching the foot with a tissue or a soft cloth. Though this may be perceived as painful at first, with repeated exposures the brain adapts and begins to respond normally to this sensory input, which means that the patient no longer perceives it as painful. Treatment progression may include exposure to rougher fabrics, brushes, sand, hot- and cold-water baths, and movements. The goal is to restore normal sensation in the painful area so that it will respond to sensory input in the same way that the other body parts do.

Passive Physical Therapy Interventions

Passive therapies include manual interventions, such as massage, as well as interventions that include the use of specialized equipment such as transcutaneous electrical nerve stimulation (TENS). These therapies can be very helpful, especially early in a PT program. But there are only limited data on their long-term effectiveness, and some passive interventions may be contraindicated for some children.

TRANSCUTANEOUS ELECTRICAL NERVE STIMULATION

A transcutaneous electrical nerve stimulation (TENS) unit may be prescribed when there is a localized area of persistent pain or discomfort. A TENS unit looks like a small box with wires attached and a small, sticky electrode connected to each wire. The electrodes are applied to the skin around the painful area. When the TENS unit is turned on it provides an electrical current that feels like a vibration on the skin. This vibratory stimulation is thought to flood the nervous system and brain with incoming sensations that essentially mask pain signals. There is often some trial and error involved in finding the optimal placement for the electrodes as well as the settings that provide the best pain relief.

Many children find benefit from TENS, though some do not like the sensation and others find it does not provide any symptom relief. For children who do find that it helps, they usually feel less pain within an hour. But the TENS unit is just a temporary fix; it is not a cure. Most people's pain returns within an hour of discontinuing its use. On the positive side, a TENS unit is small and portable and can easily be used at home or school after a PT has taught the child and parent how to use it properly. There is also very little potential for side effects from this device. For these reasons, the TENS unit can be a useful strategy for reducing in-the-moment pain, increasing comfort, and for promoting better function.

NEUROMUSCULAR ELECTRICAL STIMULATION

Neuromuscular electrical stimulation (NMES, or E-stim) is similar to TENS in that it uses a machine with wires and sticky electrodes that are applied to the skin. But E-stim uses a stronger electrical current and works by stimulating muscle contraction and relaxation in a way that is designed to mimic real muscle movements. It is used to retrain muscles, promote healing, reduce swelling, and reduce pain.

Occupational Therapy

Sometimes children with chronic pain are referred to an occupational therapy (OT) provider to help with pain. Occupational therapists are trained to analyze carefully how a child functions in his or her environment and to help make adaptive changes that can ease the pain or improve functioning. For example, a child who has pain in his wrist might be aggravating symptoms by the way he takes notes at school. An occupational therapist might suggest in this case ergonomic changes, a brace to help protect the wrist from strain, or alternative methods for note taking, such as typing. Occupational therapists also focus on helping children to feel competent with daily living tasks. For example, a child with foot pain may have trouble putting on her own sock or shoe, but an occupational therapist can show that child strategies for independently getting that sock and shoe on with the least amount of discomfort. An OT provider can also help to evaluate your child's daily activities to uncover if there are routines or daily tasks that may be unintentionally triggering a pain cycle.

♦

How to Help

1. CONSIDER PHYSICAL OR OCCUPATIONAL THERAPY

If your child has become weak from lack of activity, is fearful of engaging in activities because he or she worries about exacerbating pain or causing injury, or seems generally to be struggling with the physicality of daily tasks, talk to your doctor about whether physical therapy, occupational therapy, or both, should be considered in your child's care plan.

2. FIND A PROVIDER

Finding a caring PT or OT provider who has experience with children is essential to success with these interventions. It's also very useful if she or he has worked with people struggling to deal with chronic pain. Contact your pediatrician or primary care provider for a referral, or ask friends and family for references. You can also check "Move Forward PT," the American Physical Therapy Association's website for patients (www.moveforwardpt.com).

3. MAKE SURE YOUR PROVIDER IS A GOOD FIT FOR YOUR CHILD

Physical therapy and occupational therapy can be fun, engaging, and empowering experiences for children. But it's also a lot of work. It's important that your child is paired with a provider who is a good match and who provides a lot of encouragement and support. Your child should like her PT and OT provider, even if she may not always like what that provider suggests during therapy.

4. SUPPORT YOUR CHILD'S PHYSICAL OR OCCUPATIONAL THERAPIST

The purpose of PT and OT is to help your child move more freely and with less pain, so she can get back to the flow of her daily life. This takes work, and PT and OT providers must frequently push kids just beyond their comfort zone to get results. Make sure your child knows the possible benefits of all her hard work, and that while interventions may be difficult at times, you expect that she will try her hardest during each therapy session.

5. FOLLOW THE HOME-BASED PROGRAM

A child will usually have PT or OT sessions two or three times per week, but they can be held as infrequently as once a week or as often as every day. Generally the appointments are more frequent at the start of a PT or OT intervention and less frequent as treatment progresses. Regardless of how many times per week your child has PT or OT, there will be homework: specific stretches, exercises, or tasks that are designed to reinforce the skills learned in the guided sessions. The more consistently that kids keep up with this homework, the faster their brains will adapt to moving and functioning with less pain, so parents should make this daily practice a priority. Depending on the age and stage of your child, you might simply remind your child, actively participate (for example, by counting the repetitions of a particular exercise or assisting with desensitization), help with coping, or set up a calendar to chart his or her progress (possibly with small rewards for staying on track and reaching a goal).

8

Medications and Supplements

Medications are usually an important part of helping a child to recover from pain. But there is not a single medication that works well for everyone, and medications alone typically do not completely eliminate chronic pain. Moreover, for a significant number of children pain medications offer little benefit. For these reasons, medications, like all of the strategies I review in this book, should be part of a comprehensive, multidisciplinary approach for the management of chronic pediatric pain. It would be beyond the scope of this book to review all medications that may be used in the treatment of pediatric pain, so this section of the book focuses on the types of medications that are used to treat the most common pediatric chronic pain problems, namely headache, abdominal pain, musculoskeletal pain, and neuropathic pain.

The Art of Medication Management

Many of my physician colleagues have explained that managing pain with medication is sometimes more akin to art than science. Physicians often develop personal preferences for which medication to try first and, if that doesn't produce the desired improvement, which should be given next. Physicians may base their initial medication choices on new research they discover, clinical experience, a patient's mood or sleep disturbances, side effect or safety profiles, or other reasons. There is indeed good empirical support for the use of medications in the management of chronic pain. But there is still often an element of trial and error. There are various classes of medications that can be effective, and ranges of effectiveness for each medication. Even our most targeted pain medications do not work systematically for all children and adolescents, and all patients respond somewhat differently to the active ingredients and side effects of various medicines. Children also metabolize medication at different rates, making it hard at times to predict optimal dosages. Additionally, some medications seem to work for a while and then, for reasons we sometimes do and sometimes don't understand, stop working.

For all of these reasons obtaining the optimal medication-based therapy for an individual's pain can at times be a frustrating process for parents and kids. Yet the challenges of medication-based therapies are usually worth working through: medications can be very beneficial in the treatment of chronic pain, especially if the pain is disabling. Because medication management is more of a process and less of a "quick fix," parents need to have confidence in their prescribing physician and be informed about the use of medications for chronic pain.

Commonly Prescribed Medications for Chronic Pain

Interestingly, the types of medicines that seem to help most with chronic pain are not what people generally think of as "pain medicine." The medications that most effectively treat chronic pain are designed to directly target the nervous system: antidepressants and anticonvulsants. Both of these medications work to decrease the sensitivity of the nervous system at the level of the brain and may also modulate messages coming to and from the peripheral nervous system. Both of these classes of medication have been used safely in children, and there is clinical support for using these medications to treat chronic pain. But neither antidepressants nor anticonvulsants have been approved by the FDA for the treatment of chronic pain in children, and some of these medications can have potentially serious side effects. For this reason, a general pediatrician may not feel comfortable routinely prescribing these medications for pain. Fortunately, physicians who regularly treat chronic pain in children are very knowledgeable about the safety profiles of these medications and have a high level of comfort and confidence in prescribing and monitoring their use when they are the best option.

Because parents are frequently confused when their child is prescribed either an anticonvulsant or antidepressant for pain, it can be helpful to understand how and why each of these medications became part of the arsenal for effective pain management.

ANTICONVULSANTS

Anticonvulsants such as gabapentin (Neurontin) were first developed to treat seizures. Quite by accident, they were found to be also very useful for treating chronic pain that has a nerve-related, or neuropathic, component. Doctors often prescribe anticonvulsants for complex regional pain syndrome, fibromyalgia, and chronic headaches, among other disorders. For effectiveness, anticonvulsants require regular and consistent dosing multiple times per day; they are not used intermittently when a child experiences pain. Dosages usually start small and are often increased over several days or weeks until an effective dose is reached. Anticonvulsants are not addictive, but the body does get used to having the medication and for this reason, when a person decides to stop taking it, the dose is slowly weaned over several days or weeks to avoid the potential for uncomfortable side effects.

TRICYCLIC ANTIDEPRESSANTS

Tricyclic antidepressants (TCAs) such as amitriptyline (Elavil) and nortriptyline (Pamelor) are considered "old school" antidepressants. They were developed in the 1960s and were among the first psychopharma-cological therapies for major depressive disorder. Today these medications are seldom used to treat depression in adults, and are rarely if ever prescribed for mood-related difficulties in children. The reason is simple: they are not very good antidepressants. When used to treat mood, they require high dosages that are often linked to side effects that make the cost outweigh the benefit. But again, quite by accident, it was discovered that low doses of these medications often lead to significant improvements in chronic pain.

Parents are sometimes surprised when their child is prescribed an "antidepressant" for the treatment of pain, but the truth is that TCAs are currently used almost exclusively to treat pain. Because these medications can be used in very low doses to treat pain, there are fewer side effects to manage. Many of the mild side effects that do occur (dry mouth, fatigue, mental clouding) improve once the body adjusts to the medication in a few weeks and, much like with the anticonvulsants, many side effects can be reduced significantly by starting with a low dose of the medication and slowly increasing the dose over time. In rare instances, when a child has a preexisting abnormal heart rhythm, this class of medications can trigger irregular heart rates. For this reason, many providers require children to have a screening electrocardiogram (EKG) to rule out any risk for heart complications. This simple screening test measures a child's heart rhythms and is done by placing sticky sensor pads on a child's chest for a few minutes. The test is not at all uncomfortable for children and can often be completed in a pediatrician's office.

One particularly welcome side effect of these medications is that they temporarily make people drowsy. This can actually be a bonus. Many providers prescribe TCAs at nighttime for kids who have pain and disrupted sleep because they often provide relief from both problems. While TCAs generally have a good safety profile, parents should carefully monitor their administration since overdoses can be life-threatening for children. Additionally, a rare but dangerous condition called "serotonin syndrome" can occur when these medications are taken in combination with other medications that may also increase serotonin levels, such as medications that may be taken for anxiety or depression. For this reason, parents should be sure to inform prescribing physicians of all medications that their child is taking.

Aside from helping to reduce chronic pain and decreasing the sensitivity of the nervous system, anticonvulsants and TCAs are nonaddictive and are typically well tolerated. All medications have side effects, and one side effect of these medications is the risk of an increase in depression and suicidality. This potential risk is sometimes called "the black box warning" because it is printed on the side of many medications in a black box. Parents should know that the actual increased incidence rate for suicidality on these medications is *very* low (.002 to 1.6 percent). If your child is currently feeling depressed, however, or has a history of depression or suicidality, this should be brought to your physician's attention prior to starting a medication with a black box warning. Additionally, it is always important for parents to report significant mood changes to their child's physician whenever a child starts any new medication. (If your child is young, it may be best to have this and other discussions about side effects privately so she does not become unnecessarily alarmed.) Keep in mind that physicians would not prescribe a medication if they did not believe that the benefits outweighed any potential risks. It's also helpful for parents to consider that untreated chronic pain has a higher risk for triggering depression than does taking these medications.

Other Commonly Prescribed Medications for Pain

MUSCLE RELAXANTS

The goal of muscle relaxants is simply to reduce muscle tension or to relieve a muscle spasm. Muscle relaxants can be a useful short-term intervention for easing the chronically tense or rigid muscles that are frequently associated with musculoskeletal pain. These medications are typically prescribed to take "as needed" for managing symptoms and they work quickly, usually within an hour, to provide relief. Muscle relaxants such as cyclobenzaprine (Flexeril), tizanidine (Zanaflex), diazepam (Valium), and baclofen (Lioresal) act on the central nervous system by reducing involuntary muscle tension or rigidity, a common cause of musculoskeletal pain and discomfort. They should be used on a short-term basis, not chronically. Muscle relaxants may also be prescribed in conjunction with a physical therapy or rehabilitation program so that a person can be comfortable enough to participate in the physical activity that is needed to retrain tense or rigid muscles. Without some type of physical therapy (such as stretching, exercise, or yoga), muscles that have been chronically tight or in spasm may return to being tight or in spasm when the medication wears off. Muscle relaxants are also sometimes prescribed to help patients relax and get comfortable at night since these medications often make patients sleepy (some, such as diazepam, will reduce anxiety as well).

ANTISPASMODICS

Antispasmodics are used to reduce the abdominal spasms that are associated with irritable bowel syndrome (IBS) or functional abdominal pain (FAP). Antispasmodics such as dicyclomine (Bentyl) and hyoscyamine (Anaspaz, Cystospaz, Levsin, NuLev) reduce abdominal cramping by relaxing the smooth muscles of the gut. Similar to the muscle relaxants, antispasmodics may also generate general feelings of relaxation.

PRESCRIPTION TOPICAL TREATMENTS

Medications prescribed for topical use can be effective when pain is localized to a specific area. These medications work by delivering medicine though the top layers of the skin and are most effective when pain is neuropathic (nerve-related) and when the pain problem is closer to the surface of the skin. Topical treatments do not work well for deeper kinds of pain such as abdominal pain or headache pain, or when pain is widespread.

A big advantage to topical treatments is that they are only minimally absorbed into the bloodstream, so they tend to have far fewer side effects than oral medications can have. Additionally, topical treatments are often easy to use and don't frequently interact with other medications. Topical medications can be incorporated into a cream, lotion, gel, or patch, and they are typically applied to the skin one to four times per day. The most common topical prescriptions include either local anesthetics such as lidocaine or nonsteroidal anti-inflammatory drugs (NSAIDS) such as diclofenac (Flector Patch). Physicians can also prescribe compounded gels or creams that include other active ingredients.

Nonprescription Medications and Nutritional Supplements

There are many medications, vitamins, and therapies that are available in your local drug or health food store that may be effective for the treatment of pain. You should always let your child's doctor know if you are using these interventions—or even better, ask the doctor first to reduce the possibility that they will react with your child's prescribed medications. Generally these are safe, but even natural remedies can have side effects, so parents should also monitor carefully their child's use of any supplement.

OVER-THE-COUNTER TOPICAL PAIN RELIEVERS

Nonprescription topical creams, lotions, gels, or patches, collectively classified as "counterirritants," may provide some short-term numbing relief for sore muscles and joints or nerve irritation. Products such as Icy Hot, Tiger Balm, and Biofreeze all use menthol as their active ingredient. Menthol, when applied topically, produces a numbing sensation that can be very soothing. Over-the-counter nonsteroidal creams such as Aspercreme and Sportscreme may provide relief from minor muscle injuries or joint irritations. Generally, topical treatments have relatively few side effects and are safe to try, but there are no data on their effectiveness in treating chronic pain conditions in children. If trying these topical treatments, keep in mind that they are recommended for short-term use (seven to ten days) and should of course be discontinued if your child has any local rash or reaction to the product.

PROBIOTICS

Probiotics are actually live bacterial microorganisms. Over the past twenty years clinical studies have established that probiotic therapy can be beneficial in treating several gastrointestinal disorders in children, including symptoms of ulcerative colitis and Crohn's disease. Specifically, probiotic therapy seems to reduce diarrhea, gas, and bloating. The microorganisms found in most probiotics naturally occur in the lining of the gut, so they are widely thought to be safe. In the United States, however, most probiotics do not undergo FDA testing so there is no way to be sure which ingredients are in the supplement. Because different strains of probiotics may be more or less effective at treating a particular symptom, you should consult your child's provider to determine what type of probiotic may be the best option.

VITAMIN SUPPLEMENTS

While a well-balanced diet helps to ensure that children and adolescents get necessary vitamins, some vitamin supplements may offer additional benefits for children with chronic pain. Parents should talk with their child's doctor before starting any individual vitamin supplementation program.

Vitamin D

Vitamin D is naturally produced in the body when our skin is exposed to the sun. About 85 percent of our required vitamin D can be obtained with relatively minimal daily sun exposure (just ten to thirty minutes). Vitamin D can also be absorbed from eating fish and fortified foods such as milk and cereal. Low vitamin D, which most commonly occurs in the winter or when there is limited outdoor activity, can be associated with fatigue and muscle pain. If your child has low levels (ask your doctor to check if you are unsure), a vitamin D supplement can be an important part of your child's pain-management plan.

Riboflavin (Vitamin B2)

The vitamin riboflavin naturally occurs in milk, meat, eggs, nuts, enriched flour, and many green vegetables, and most people can easily obtain the recommended daily requirements with a balanced diet. When B2 supplements are taken in higher doses, however, they have been linked to reduced frequency of migraines in adults. There are few side effects, but the positive effects are not usually noticeable until after about three months of treatment, so it's important to take this vitamin for several months to ascertain if it will be beneficial.

Coenzyme Q-10 (CoQ-10)

Coenzyme Q-10 occurs naturally in our bodies and is partly responsible for providing energy to cells throughout the body. Some studies have shown the supplement to be helpful for counteracting fatigue, low energy, and migraine headache. In children, it's been found to decrease the frequency of migraine headache by as much as 30 percent. Similar to vitamin B2, it can take several months before the benefits are fully attained.

Omega 3's

Omega 3's are the healthy fats that are naturally found in foods such as fish and flax seed. Fish oil supplements are also a good resource for Omega 3's. Omega 3's are noted for reducing inflammation throughout the body, and because reduced inflammation leads to reduced pain for a variety of pain problems, Omega 3 supplements may offer benefit to a wide range of painful conditions.

HERBAL TREATMENTS

Herbal treatments have been used for centuries to treat common pain problems such as headache, joint pain, and abdominal pain. In Western medicine, even though many modern pharmaceutical companies use compounds originally derived from herbs or modeled after the active ingredients in plants or flowers, herbal supplements have not been widely prescribed. But this seems to be changing. In Europe as many as half of physicians prescribe herbal remedies, and the practice is becoming more popular in the United States as well. This is likely due to an increase in medical research evidence demonstrating the benefits of some herbal treatments. Though the body of scientific evidence remains small, a growing number of positive double-blind placebo controlled research trials (the gold standard for testing effectiveness in medicine) are shedding a promising light on a handful of potentially effective herbal remedies. Caution is still needed, however: while there are many herbal supplements on the market, only a few pass the test of being empirically supported (these are mentioned below), and different preparations have different herbal strengths. More importantly, while herbal supplements are natural, they can still have side effects, interact with other pharmaceuticals, and be toxic. For these reasons, parents should always talk to their child's doctor before using herbal supplements.

Melatonin

Chronic pain frequently interferes with sleep. Restoring sleep can help the body to heal, reset the signaling pathways of the nervous system, improve mood, and increase a sense of well-being. There are many behavioral strategies that can help to restore sleep (see Chapter 17 for suggestions). But melatonin can offer additional support as a useful short-term strategy when sleep is disrupted. Melatonin is a naturally occurring hormone that is secreted by the pineal gland in the brain when the eyes are exposed to darkness. Many animals (and plants) naturally produce melatonin and its purpose is to gently ease the body into sleep. Although it is a naturally occurring hormone and has a good safety profile, it is not recommended that children or adolescents take melatonin long-term. When taken for longer periods of time, there is increased risk for side effects such as low mood and stomach irritation, and its

long-term effects, if any, on childhood development are not well understood. For this reason, children and adolescents should take the small-
est dose of melatonin that seems beneficial and use it only for short
periods of time.

Butterbur

Butterbur is a Chinese herb that has been found to reduce inflammation. It's been used to treat a wide range of pain problems including
migraine headache, stomach pain, and joint or muscle pain. It's also
suggested that it may help to reduce anxiety, improve depression, and
treat insomnia. To date, research suggests that it is most effective for
migraine prevention and treatment, though a small body of evidence
suggests improvements with various other types of pain.

A word of caution: some herbal supplements such as Butterbur may
contain pyrrolizidine alkaloids (PAs), which are produced by plants
as a natural insect repellent and are highly toxic to human livers. It
is essential to find Chinese herbs such as Butterbur that are certified
"PA free."

Feverfew (Parthenolide)

Feverfew is a daisy-like plant that originated in Bulgaria but now thrives
in much of Eastern Europe. It has been used for centuries to treat fevers, joint pain, and headache. Current research supports only its use
for reducing the frequency of migraine headaches.

Peppermint Oil

Peppermint oil has gained popularity in pediatrics over the past ten
years for its effectiveness in reducing pain associated with recurrent
abdominal pain and irritable bowel syndrome. It's also been found to
reduce nausea. The natural menthol in peppermint oil is believed to
reduce muscle contractions, resulting in less frequent and less intense
abdominal spasms. It's also thought that peppermint oil may reduce gas
and stimulate digestion.

Medications Not Commonly Used for Chronic Pain

Over-the-counter pain relievers such as acetaminophen (Tylenol) or ibuprofen (Advil or Motrin) are safe and effective for treating a child's short-term pain. In some cases, however, these commonly used medications can make pain problems worse over the long term. For example, acetaminophen can be useful for occasional headache pain, but can cause more frequent and intense "rebound" headaches if taken regularly over many weeks or months. Without realizing it, people can create or reinforce a cycle of pain; more headache pain can spur patients to reach for more acetaminophen, and frequent use of acetaminophen can lead to more painful headaches. Similarly, while ibuprofen can be useful for reducing inflammation and pain in the short-term, when taken over longer periods of time it can lead to gastrointestinal irritation, diarrhea, reflux, and stomach pain. For these reasons, these common pain-relieving medications are usually recommended for intermittent use only and not for daily, long-term management of chronic pain.

Another major category of "pain medicines" includes prescription narcotic or opioid medications. This class of medicines reduces pain by broadly dulling nervous system activity, and can be highly effective. Doctors commonly prescribe opioids for acute pain that is expected to resolve within a few days or weeks—for instance, post-surgical pain, pain from a recent injury, or an acute flare of disease-related pain. Opioids can be very effective at masking pain and so give the body a chance to heal, which is very important in these situations. Opioids have been proven safe to use for short-term or acute pain management and parents should not be afraid to have their children take an opioid prescribed by a physician.

If pain has become a chronic problem, however, opioids are rarely a wise choice for several important reasons. First, many patients build up a tolerance to opioids. This means that higher and higher doses are required to get the same pain-management effect, and so the likelihood of negative side effects—like nausea and constipation, but also sleepiness, reduced emotional sensitivity, and sluggish cognition—increases as well. Second, the risk for opioid misuse and opioid poisoning is significant. Young children can have life-threatening side effects from even a relatively small overdose and older children can also experience serious side effects from unintentional overdosing. Teenagers have the added risk of potentially misusing the medication or giving it to peers for recreational purposes. For these reasons, when opioids are prescribed, parents should adhere to the following precautions: (1) always keep opioid medications in a locked cabinet and be especially sure they are out of reach of younger children, (2) maintain good communication if multiple caregivers (such as parents, grandparents, and a babysitter) are administering the medication to a child and be sure that anyone who is administering the medication is educated about how to do so properly, (3) only fill opioid prescriptions from a single medical provider, and (4) properly dispose of unused opioid medications to reduce the risk for accidental ingestion, diversion, or abuse.

Beyond the risks for tolerance and misuse, opioids are not generally a good choice for persistent pain because they don't actually help to improve the problem; they simply mask it. Recall that once a pain problem has become chronic, the actual hardware in the body has generally healed as much as it's going to heal. At this point, it's a nervous system, or software, problem. Opioids do not help restore the nervous system "software." Moreover, they have numerous side effects that can impair a child's ability to get through a typical day and can induce feelings of depression, making it increasingly difficult for children to get back on track with school or daily activities.

Other Medically Based Treatment Options

This chapter offers a broad overview of some of the most commonly prescribed medications for the treatment of pain. It is by no means a comprehensive review of all of the medications or supplements that are used for pain. Beyond the medications and supplements in this chapter, there may be other medical interventions, such as nerve blocks (to take just one example), that may be of medical benefit in some cases. A review of all medical interventions that may be indicated for the treatment of pain, however, is beyond the scope of this book, in part because every child's pain presentation requires a thoughtful and individualized approach by a knowledgeable provider or team of providers. Parents are encouraged to remain open to learning about why particular medications, supplements, or medical interventions either are or are not recommended for inclusion in their child's care plan.

◆

How to Help

1. ESTABLISH A RELATIONSHIP WITH A KNOWLEDGEABLE PHYSICIAN

Find a pain-management physician or a specialist with whom you feel you can collaborate to improve your child's health. You should feel that your child's doctor really listens and understands the challenges your child faces and has answered your questions about medication management. Establish an ongoing communication plan with your child's physician; whether that involves checking in with nurses or contacting your child's doctor directly will vary by provider.

2. MONITOR YOUR CHILD'S MEDICATIONS

Children and adolescents need a parent to monitor their medications to be sure they are taking the prescribed dose in the prescribed way. This is especially important when starting a medication or changing a dosing schedule. If children aren't taking the medicine as prescribed, it is very difficult to determine whether it is effective. Inconsistently timed dosages, too, can make side effects more difficult to tolerate. As a general rule, an adult should lock up all medications when not dispensing them, especially TCAs and opioids that have a high rate of toxicity if taken incorrectly or misused. All parents should closely monitor the use of opioid medications to reduce the risk of unintended overdoses as well as the chance of diversion for recreational use, and when children no longer require opioids, parents are urged to properly dispose of any unused medications to reduce the future possibility of misuse or abuse. If your older adolescent would like to independently manage his or her nonopioid medications, this transition should be done gradually and with continued parental oversight.

3. REPORT SIDE EFFECTS

When starting a new medication or changing a dose, notify your child's prescribing doctor immediately if there are any side effects, including changes in mood or behavior, that are disruptive or of concern. Some mild side effects can wear off after the body adjusts or acclimates to a new medication, but you should always contact your child's doctor if new or unusual symptoms emerge when starting a new medication. If for any reason you decide to discontinue a medication, talk to your doctor—don't just stop administering it to your child. Many medications used for pain management need to be slowly weaned to avoid unpleasant side effects, and your doctor can help in this process.

4. BE PATIENT

Medications used for the treatment of chronic pain can take several weeks to reach their full effectiveness, and return doctor's visits for medication management may only occur every six to eight weeks. Give the medicine time to work before abandoning the effort. And let your child know that although he or she may feel better in a few days, for some children it takes longer for the medications to be fully effective.

5. TELL YOUR CHILD'S DOCTOR ABOUT ANY OVER-THE-COUNTER MEDICATIONS, VITAMINS, OR HERBAL SUPPLEMENTS

"Natural" remedies, including those listed in this chapter, can also have side effects and may not work well in combination with prescribed medications. Be sure your child's doctor knows about all of your child's medications and supplements.

6. MEDICATIONS AND SUPPLEMENTS:
ONLY PART OF THE SOLUTION

It's easy to get caught up in the hope that a medication or supplement will be the answer to a child's chronic pain problem. But medication alone is seldom the answer. It is more reasonable to expect that a medication will reduce the frequency and intensity of symptoms. Approaching medication and supplement use as part of a comprehensive pain-management program will help you to set appropriate expectations for your child and your entire family. Be sure to communicate this expectation clearly with your child so she understands that medications are only part of the solution.

9

Additional Interventions

The gold-standard treatments for pain management, including behavioral medicine, structured physical or occupational therapy, and medication, have decades of data supporting their effectiveness in the treatment of chronic pain in children. Providers stand by these approaches because they work well for the majority of children and so should be among the first strategies tried. But there is more that can be done.

Adding on to a pain-management plan with additional interventions can serve to enhance outcomes and in many cases increase a child's experience of comfort. It's important for parents both to consider the pros and cons of each strategy and to discuss possible interventions with a child's primary provider or pain-management specialist. In many cases, getting input from your child can also boost his willingness to participate.

You can think of the interventions in this chapter as a sort of intervention pyramid. The top-tier strategies are tried and true. Your child may not need all of these strategies, but if they are recommended for your child, you should jump in with confidence. Second-tier strategies are considered safe to try, but have less research supporting their effectiveness. Third-tier strategies have the lowest ratio of success and also may have an element of risk or harm associated with them; parents should use caution if considering these interventions. Keep in mind that not every child needs every service or intervention, and in some cases, more intervention is not always better. As with all approaches in pain management, balance is key. Consulting with one of your child's doctors is essential for sorting out which additional interventions may be useful for your child and in what order they should be tried.

Top-Tier Interventions

In addition to the trifecta of services that are typically included in a multidisciplinary pain-management team—namely, behavioral therapy, structured physical or occupational therapy, and medications—there are a number of other interventions that can be enormously helpful in coping with chronic pain and pain-related difficulties. Below are some of the most highly recommended, top-tier rated interventions that dovetail well with many pain-management plans.

ACUPUNCTURE

Acupuncture is a traditional Chinese medicine that has been practiced for thousands of years. The practice is based on the premise that emotional or physical discomfort is the result of an unbalanced life force, called qi ("chee"), which is believed to flow through meridians, or pathways, in the body. Acupuncture is the practice of placing very thin needles into identified points along the meridians to help improve the flow, or balance, of one's life force. The science of acupuncture is still not well understood, but in Western medicine it is generally believed that the placement of needles in the acupuncture points may improve blood flow in muscles and connective tissues and trigger our nervous system to release natural analgesics, or painkillers.

Research on acupuncture suggests that it often alleviates a variety of different pain symptoms, including headache, menstrual pain, fibromyalgia, back pain, joint pain, abdominal pain, and a variety of nerve- or muscle-based pain conditions. It has also demonstrated benefit for insomnia, anxiety, and poor concentration. Although most research on acupuncture has focused on the adult population and not children, acupuncture is widely accepted as a safe treatment, and a growing number of pediatric providers endorse its use for their patients. That said, if a child is fearful of acupuncture, anxiety about the procedure could outweigh the potential benefit.

At the first acupuncture session, the provider will gather detailed information about a person's pain problem as well as information about his or her general health and well-being. The treatment involves resting on a table while the provider inserts between five to twenty needles. The inserted needles are sometimes stimulated with heat or with movement, such as turning, to increase their effectiveness. Needles are placed at the area of discomfort, and are also commonly placed in other areas such as ears, forehead, wrists, hands, and feet. Once inserted, the needles remain in place for ten to twenty minutes. It's important to note that the needles used in acupuncture are very different from the kinds of needles used for vaccines or to draw blood. Needles used to administer medication or draw blood need to be hollow and firm so as to puncture the skin and allow for the administration or withdrawal of fluid. In contrast, acupuncture needles are very thin and flexible. They cause minimal damage to the skin and there is rarely any blood at the insertion site. Most people do not find the needles painful, and some people do not feel them at all. When the insertion of the needle is felt, it is frequently described as a tinge of discomfort that resolves quickly. Recipients usually remain clothed throughout the treatment, unless the area of discomfort is not easily accessible through clothing. Typically a child will know within three sessions if acupuncture is helping his or her pain. A course of acupuncture can range from six to twelve sessions and the cost is typically $75–95 for the intake (history-taking) session and $50–70 for treatments.

Reports of adverse side effects as a result of acupuncture are very rare and the risk for most patients is minimal. Because of the invasive nature of acupuncture, it is generally a well-regulated practice: parents should ensure that any provider they identify is certified. Interestingly, a small but growing number of physicians who specialize in pain management are becoming certified in acupuncture and are integrating this into their medical practice. Working with a physician who administers acupuncture can mean that the treatments are covered by insurance.

For those who would like to try acupuncture but are needle phobic, there is a related practice called acupressure, which uses healing pressure, rather than needles, at specific acupuncture points. Acupressure may be an appealing option to children because it is noninvasive, though unfortunately its effectiveness is less well established.

PSYCHIATRY

A psychiatric evaluation can be very useful if your child is struggling with persistent or impairing anxiety, depression, attention issues, or other mental health concerns. A pediatric psychiatrist may be able to offer a more individualized combination of medicines as well as careful monitoring of your child's response to those medications. The informed input of a child psychiatrist can be an important part of a pain-management plan for children who have acute or persistent symptoms of anxiety, depression, or other mental health issues.

Psychiatric services typically are covered by insurance. Most psychiatrists will meet with patients one to two times a month during the initial phase of treatment; once a child is stable with a medication, appointments may occur only every two to three months.

PROFESSIONAL ASSISTANCE WITH NUTRITION

A pediatric nutritionist specializes in helping children and families make balanced and healthy food choices to benefit their physical and emotional well-being and to promote optimal growth and development. A nutrition consultation can be especially important for children with gastrointestinal symptoms such as irritable bowel syndrome, functional abdominal pain, and chronic nausea, or for children with dietary restrictions such as celiac disease, multiple food allergies, or food intolerance. These children are at increased risk for developing irregular eating habits and may restrict their diets in an effort to alleviate symptoms—but children avoiding multiple foods may be at risk for vitamin, mineral, and macronutrient deficiencies which can prolong or exacerbate pain symptoms.

Changes in weight can also be a reason for a referral to a nutrition specialist. Whether due to medications, inactivity, stress, or poor eating habits, it is not uncommon for children to have weight changes during a time of chronic pain. Weight gain in children is important to address because it may predispose children to be overweight as adults, may interfere with rehabilitation goals if it makes children less active, and can lead to lower self-esteem. Weight loss, or a failure to gain weight, can be equally concerning. When children are underweight or are not growing as expected, they may be missing the essential nutrients necessary to heal and to think clearly, feel chronically cold or fatigued, and be prone to sleep disturbances.

The designation "nutritionist" may be used even if a provider has not obtained specialized training or is self-taught. Parents need to look specifically for a "registered dietary nutritionist" (RDN) to ensure they are getting the services of a trained, credentialed professional. Depending on what state you live in, many dietitians will also be licensed by the state. To find a licensed dietitian/nutritionist (LDN) for your child, ask your pediatrician for a recommendation or search the website of the Academy of Nutrition and Dietetics: www.eatright.org/programs/rdnfinder.

It is helpful to find a provider who is positive, who helps families make manageable changes in diets and eating routines, and who is careful not to blame either parents or children along the way. While some nutritionists may make recommendations and then consider the treatment complete, parents can often request to have their child seen again in a few weeks for a follow-up session. Additional visits can help to hold parents and kids accountable for making positive and lasting changes.

SLEEP ANALYSIS

Disrupted sleep, whether due to difficulty falling asleep or problems staying asleep, is perhaps the most common problem associated with chronic pain. Many sleep problems can be addressed with behavior interventions at home (see Chapter 17). But while chronic pain certainly leads to poor sleep, it is also true that poor sleep can be a root cause of chronic pain. If sleep disruptions preceded your child's pain problem, if your child snores so loudly that you can hear it in another room, or if primary sleep disorders such as narcolepsy, sleep walking, or restless leg syndrome run in your family, you should talk to your child's doctor about the possibility of doing a sleep study.

A pediatric sleep study usually involves a multidisciplinary team that includes pediatric specialists from fields such as psychology, pulmonology, otolaryngology, and nutrition. A sleep study may involve an overnight stay in a sleep lab during which a child's sleep is observed and monitored via sensors placed on his or her head and body. Sleep studies can sometimes be completed at home with portable equipment and sometimes recommendations can even be made without the need to do an overnight sleep study.

Second-Tier Interventions

The interventions in this section have been found to provide benefit for children with pain, though the research literature that supports them is more limited than that for the top-tier therapies. Some of these interventions may have lower rates of success or just have yet to accumulate a strong body of empirical evidence. Importantly, none of these interventions are thought to be harmful and so are good choices for kids to try, especially in combination with top-tier treatments.

YOGA

Yoga is the practice of combining breathing exercises with different postures designed to improve mindfulness, stress level, and flexibility. Yoga is a well-tolerated practice for patients with chronic pain because it can be adapted to all skill levels. Iyengar yoga is a specific type of yoga that focuses on the therapeutic alignment of muscles, bones, and joints and emphasizes rehabilitation. Iyengar yoga uses blankets, bolsters, and other props to make the practice comfortable and safe for people who may have limited movement due to pain or disability. Yoga may offer benefit on several fronts: the stretching and strengthening can support general conditioning, the integrated breathing exercises can help with relaxation, and the group setting can be a welcoming way to join with others around healing.

Yoga has been studied in a variety of clinical areas in adults and the results have been generally positive. Pediatric research on yoga is limited, but some studies have shown clinical benefit in children with disease-related pain such as rheumatoid arthritis and functional pain such as irritable bowel syndrome. For this reason, yoga is commonly recommended as a helpful intervention.

AROMATHERAPY

Aromatherapy is the practice of using essential oils, typically derived from the leaves or roots of flowers and plants, to soothe, relax, or stimulate the body. The practice of aromatherapy has been around since the early 1900s and involves identifying scents and application methods that a person finds helpful or soothing. Ultimately every individual decides for himself or herself what works best to reduce symptoms. Once a person determines which essential oil scents are beneficial, the oils can be mixed with lotions or alcohol bases and can be used in a variety of ways including being rubbed directly into the skin, sprayed into the air, used in a massage oil, or simply inhaled.

There is some consensus in the field of aromatherapy that certain scents are consistently linked to specific benefits. For example, lavender is thought to produce feelings of relaxation, eucalyptus to reduce headache, and lemon or orange to reduce nausea. Aromatherapy is hypothesized to work by stimulating olfactory nerves in the nose that connect to the emotion centers of the brain, resulting in a calming or soothing effect of the nervous system. This is an unproven hypothesis, but given what we know about the mind-body connection, it's not unreasonable to think that certain scents may be connected to comfort and relaxation for some people. Recall from Chapter 2 that the memory and emotion centers of the brain help to decode sensory signals (like the scent of a cake baking in the oven) and can thus trigger positive feelings.

The success of aromatherapy may be due in part to the power of suggestion and the soothing environment that is often created as part of the practice. The science of aromatherapy is limited and results are mixed. One recent randomized, controlled study found that children who were exposed to lavender aromatherapy following a tonsillectomy required less acetaminophen after their surgery as compared to children who were not exposed to lavender. Several other recent studies have found that while parents and children reported having less distress while using aromatherapy, there was not a statistically significant decrease in the intensity or frequency of pain.

Aromatherapy can be provided by an "aromatherapy consultant," but it is also a safe and easy intervention to try on your own at home. Simply visit a natural foods store with your child to test various scents. One helpful and fun strategy to try is to pair a favorite aromatherapy scent with a favorite relaxation practice (see Part 3 for relaxation strategies). Over time, the brain may associate the scent with the state of relaxation so that your child will be able to trigger a state of relaxation just by smelling that particular scent. One word of caution with aromatherapy: younger children should be warned that these scents are for external use only and could be dangerous if swallowed.

REIKI

Reiki is an alternative healing technique with Japanese roots that is promoted as a way to reduce stress, increase relaxation, and encourage healing. During a Reiki session, a practitioner will gently place his or her hands on the patient in order to foster the flow of an unseen "life force energy." Reiki is based on the theory that when people have a low "life force energy" they are more likely to be sick or stressed. Conversely, when "life force energy" is high, people feel emotional and physical well-being.

Reiki is considered a safe practice with no identified side effect. It is ranked here as a second-tier treatment, however, because placebo-controlled research trials have never shown that Reiki is any more effective than a placebo. In other words, while some people report that Reiki is helpful, there are no data to back up the claim that Reiki promotes healing or reduces pain beyond standard relaxation practices. Additionally, Reiki is a passive intervention. In other words, children can't do this for themselves. Thus, while children may experience "in-the-moment" comfort, it may be hard to re-create these feelings outside of the Reiki session.

A child receiving a Reiki treatment will stretch out on a bed or exam table, fully clothed, in a comfortable position. Sometimes children are asked to hold a crystal or the provider places a crystal under an area of discomfort. Often there is soft, relaxing music playing in the background and the provider may use strategies such as guided imagery to help a child relax (for more on guided imagery, see Chapter 11). The practice of Reiki itself involves having a provider place his or her hands gently on the child, or in some cases just above the child, to help improve the flow of the life force energy. Children and adolescents generally know after one session if they enjoy Reiki and want to return. Some providers suggest that a child try two or three sessions before they decide if it has helped them to feel better. Sessions can range in length from thirty to sixty minutes and are not usually covered by insurance. The cost of Reiki can vary widely, but typical sessions cost between $35 to $100.

Some patients enjoy the positive spiritual framework of Reiki and find it to be a source of comfort and healing. But there are several things that parents should be cautious of before initiating Reiki. First and foremost, the practice of Reiki is not yet well regulated. Because it is considered a "spiritual intervention," some states require that practitioners obtain an ordained minister's license before offering the service. Because Reiki is also considered a "touch therapy" some states require that practitioners obtain a license in massage therapy. Other states do not regulate Reiki practice at all. Because the field is not yet well regulated by state licensure committees it is often hard to determine how experienced or qualified a provider is. One good bet would be a local hospital or rehab center that is integrating Reiki into its palliative and pain service programs, because its practitioners would probably be licensed health care providers like nurses. Finding a reputable referral from a major medical institution is also a good option.

MASSAGE THERAPY

Massage therapy is a somewhat generic term used to describe any hands-on approach to manipulating soft tissues in the body, including muscles, tendons, and ligaments. The general goal of massage therapy is to loosen or stretch areas of the body that are tight or painful. There are many types, or "modalities," of massage, and research on massage does not generally differentiate between different modalities.

Preliminary evidence shows that massage therapy is an effective treatment for adults struggling with back pain, neck pain, and widespread body pain. Broadly speaking, massage has been shown to temporarily reduce chronic pain and possibly to counter fatigue. The results, however, have not been documented to be lasting. This means that massage can be a useful intervention for providing "in-the-moment" comfort, but treatments must continue in order to maintain this benefit. It is possible that when combined with other treatment modalities such as physical therapy, the beneficial results of massage may be longer lasting. Within pediatrics, research on the effectiveness of massage for chronic pain is scarce. A few smaller case studies suggest that children report less distress, more comfort, and improved mood immediately after receiving a massage, but there is no clear research supporting longer-term benefits.

Forty-four states in the United States regulate massage therapy, but training standards vary considerably between states. There are few risks associated with massage when it is administered by a licensed and knowledgeable provider. But there are some important precautions to take if you are considering the use of massage for pain management.

If your child has an underlying medical condition, make certain that an identified massage therapist is knowledgeable about the condition before initiating treatment. It's also essential that any massage therapist working with a child has experience in pediatrics. A pediatric massage therapist will know, for example, that while it is traditional for adults to disrobe for a massage, this is not true for children—they should never be asked to take their clothing off for a massage treatment (children often instead dress in loose-fitting athletic clothes). Be aware, too, that in many states the law requires that a parent remain in the room during a massage of a minor, and even if your state does not, you should do so, for your child's safety and so you can help your child communicate to the provider any concerns or questions about the treatment.

Massage therapy is not typically covered by insurance, though many physical therapists incorporate massage into their treatment and under these circumstances it is generally covered. The national average for the cost of a massage is $60 an hour, though massages tend to be more expensive in cities and the setting of the massage (such as in a health club, spa, or wellness center) can influence the price as well.

It's important for parents to discuss with their child's providers whether massage would be a useful intervention for their child. In some circumstances massage therapy may be contraindicated; for example, if there is any chance that the massage could exacerbate an existing pain condition. But if muscle tension is a contributing factor to a child's pain condition, many providers will readily encourage the use of massage.

Third-Tier Interventions

The strategies that are identified here as "third tier" have insufficient clinical research to support their effectiveness for treating chronic pain in children. Moreover, a few of these strategies may have negative or harmful effects. For these reasons, *these treatments are not routinely recommended by pain-management specialists.*

The interventions listed in this section should be viewed with a healthy dose of skepticism. Parents are encouraged to be very cautious of interventions that are costly, have low rates of success, may have adverse effects, are performed by nonlicensed providers, or are not widely recommended by your child's medical team. Keep in mind that some alternative therapies can unfortunately lead to more disability or longer-term problems.

CRANIOSACRAL THERAPY

Craniosacral therapy is a manipulation technique based on the belief that there are small, rhythmic motions in the cranial bones that control cerebrospinal fluid pressure and arterial pressure. A craniosacral therapist applies pressure to the head, neck, and spine to manipulate these bones, which theoretically changes fluid pressures and helps to reduce various pain problems.

It is recommended that parents take great caution before taking their child to a craniosacral therapist. There is no confirmed science behind the theory of craniosacral therapy in adults or children and there is no regulation or oversight of practitioners. The manipulation of cranial bones, though intended to be gentle, remains a particularly concerning practice in pediatrics where young bodies and brains are continuing to grow and develop. For these reasons, medical professionals do not typically recommend or refer patients for craniosacral treatment.

CHIROPRACTIC THERAPY

Chiropractic therapy consists of adjusting and manipulating the neck, spine, and surrounding tissue to treat spinal subluxations, which are the hypothesized cause of a wide range of problems ranging from pain to asthma to ear infections. Chiropractors manipulate and adjust the spine using pressure, twists, stretches, and other hands-on manipulations. Most pediatric providers advise against chiropractic interventions. First, there is very little research supporting the benefit of chiropractic intervention in pediatrics. And second, while few serious adverse events have been reported in the literature, minor injuries are thought to be more prevalent (and underreported). In addition, there is concern in the medical community that taking a child to a chiropractor for pain symptoms can dangerously delay or interrupt medical evaluation and treatment.

Despite limited support from the medical and scientific community, chiropractic treatment of children is growing in popularity. Although some pediatric patients have found relief via chiropractic therapy, parents are generally cautioned against this treatment, especially for children under the age of sixteen.

HOMEOPATHY

Homeopathy is the practice of treating symptoms using highly diluted mixtures of substances such as plants, insects, or animals. The mixtures, which may be so diluted that they do not even contain trace amounts of the "active" ingredient, can be delivered as sugar pills that dissolve under the tongue, tinctures, or topical treatments. Homeopathy was developed in Germany about two hundred years ago and is based in part on the theory that lower doses of active ingredients lead to greater effectiveness. Unfortunately, systematic research and reviews of the literature do not back up this claim. To date, there is no rigorous clinical evidence to support homeopathy as an effective treatment for any specific condition. Still, the practice of homeopathy has been rapidly increasing in popularity with close to one million parents reporting that they have used homeopathy to treat their children in 2012.

Laws regulating the practice of homeopathy in the United States vary considerably by state; in some states, providers are required to be licensed health care professionals (that is, physicians, nurses, or osteopaths), while in other states unlicensed providers can practice homeopathy. Most homeopathic treatments are thought to be safe because they are almost entirely composed of water, alcohol, and sweeteners; some solutions, however, may contain metals such as mercury or iron and so potentially harm recipients, especially children. The FDA does not typically evaluate these solutions for either safety or effectiveness.

Homeopathy is inherently difficult to study with empirical research because the process is highly individualized, the practice is based on solutions that may not contain any identifiable active ingredients, and there is wide variability among providers' preparations. Homeopathic treatments can be very costly and with little science to back up this intervention, parents are advised to use other treatment modalities instead.

◆

How to Help

1. MAKE TOP-TIER INTERVENTIONS THE PRIORITY

While there are individual differences in terms of who responds best to which type of intervention, the top-tier strategies reviewed in this chapter—along with behavioral therapy, physical or occupational therapy, and medications—are proven to work across many types of pain problems and for many age groups. Pain-management specialists put a lot of confidence in these strategies because they are familiar with the research showing their effectiveness and because they see firsthand how these strategies can work with their patients. Parents should invest most of their pain-management resources in top-tier strategies. Only once these are in place should parents and kids, if they wish, explore other safe but less proven approaches that may be of interest.

2. EVALUATE AS YOU GO

Sometimes I see families who have tried a strategy like acupuncture for six months without any benefit, but continue to go to sessions with the hope that it will soon help. Yes there is good evidence for acupuncture, but acupuncture is one of those approaches that should show a benefit within a few sessions if it is going to make a meaningful difference. If it's not working by then, it's okay to try something else instead.

By contrast, I sometimes meet families who have abandoned interventions prematurely. Parents might say, "We tried one session of cognitive behavioral therapy, but my daughter didn't like it so we didn't return." Some strategies, like cognitive behavioral therapy, do take several weeks or months before benefits are noted. How can a parent know how long is too long for trying a new approach? Simply ask your child's providers. And even if the strategy seems to be working, be sure to keep the conversation going to assess if changes are needed along the way.

3. BE WARY OF QUICK FIXES

Much as we would like to find a quick fix for a child's chronic pain, it is seldom possible. As a general rule, the longer a child has been in pain, the longer it takes to undo the chronic pain problem. Any provider who is a specialist in pain management knows that getting better and learning to manage chronic pain is a process, and that lasting improvements generally unfold over weeks or months, not hours or days. Parents can help their child avoid disappointment and frustration by making sure that expectations are realistic, and by preparing the entire family for more of a marathon, rather than a sprint, toward pain management. It can be helpful for parents to track a child's progress over time so you can all see forward movement, even if it is slower than hoped, and to applaud your child's efforts to engage in a variety of treatment strategies.

4. KEEP TALKING TO YOUR CHILD'S PROVIDERS

You should always inform your child's primary provider or specialist about the treatments or interventions your child is using. Most providers are open to a wide range of treatments including alternative or complementary strategies, so don't hold back this important information. It's difficult for any provider to make an effective treatment plan if he or she is in the dark about ongoing therapies or services, and you'll want an expert's support as you coordinate all the elements of your child's recovery plan.

Part III

Reset: Moving Forward with Relaxation and Mindfulness

Most of the strategies presented in this section are rooted in techniques that have been around for thousands of years. Even more impressive, when they have been studied with the use of rigorous modern research protocols at major medical institutions around the world, the results have been crystal clear: they really work. Not only do they reduce the subjective experience of pain, but when tested with functional imaging studies, there is also evidence to show that the brain changes physiologically in response to these strategies. Some research now supports the claim that for some children and adolescents these types of skills can be even more effective than medication for restoring function and reducing pain. These highly effective strategies can be very quick to learn and none have side effects. I know it seems almost too good to be true, but these strategies really are some of the win-win approaches to pain management.

Many parents bring their child to see me for treatment because they want their child to learn relaxation strategies for managing pain. This makes my job easy. Even if a child is resistant to the idea of relaxation, having parents on board means that what I teach in my session will likely be reinforced at home, and this in turn helps to foster progress.

Other parents, however, bring their child to see me only out of due diligence. Their child's medical doctor referred them for treatment and told them it will help, but they have serious doubts that any of the mind-body approaches will be useful. Like all parents, they are desperate for quick relief for their child. I once had a father sit in my office and implore me to "put the good word in" with one of the anesthesiologists I work with to see if I could get her to prescribe stronger medications or, mercifully, do a procedure that would numb the painful area, even if the numbing medicine would only help his daughter for a day, an hour, or just five minutes. This parent was begging for something, *anything,* to bring his child immediate relief from pain. Though I knew in this case that no amount of lobbying would sway the anesthesiologist toward more medication or injections, I learned a lot from this father's earnest plea. What he was saying was: "I need a way to help reduce my daughter's suffering right *now.*" This I can tackle.

Pain can be relentless. It can feel unending. It can seem insurmountable. It can be hard for parents, much less kids, to truly buy into the fact that mind-body strategies can help to change the experience of pain, regardless of how the pain problem started. Sometimes we are drawn to the false idea that modern Western medicine is the one and only answer; or perhaps our expectation is that it is simply the most expeditious one. But it's simply not true. When I work with parents to teach them how to help their child with relaxation, I start by first acknowledging that it's okay to be skeptical. It's not uncommon for parents to think that these strategies will have little impact, are not long-term solutions, or won't work quickly enough. Understanding the science behind these strategies can help.

Recall that pain and stress can trigger our autonomic nervous system and cause an increased heart rate, shallow breathing, sweating, and feelings of uneasiness. This nervous system arousal amplifies pain signals and can make our bodies more sensitive to sensory input. Fortunately, our body has an antidote to this. It's called the parasympathetic response. You can think of the parasympathetic response as the "all clear" signal. Our brain naturally triggers the parasympathetic antidote when it believes the threat, danger, or stress has sufficiently subsided.

If the pain is persistent, or if pain-related stress is chronic, then the threat or danger remains present and the brain never sends the "all clear" signal. That means your child will be stuck in a state of high autonomic arousal. Feeling lousy. Just waiting for the "all clear." The relaxation strategies in this section of the book are a way to override the autonomic system to achieve that longed-for sense of relief. The state of relaxation is incompatible with autonomic arousal. This means that if a person can persuade the body to relax by using specific tried-and-true techniques, the brain will get the all clear signal, and both pain and stress can begin to subside.

Parents need to remind themselves often that there is indeed something very effective they can do to help ease their child's suffering for five, ten, twenty minutes or more. And the best part is that a child can learn to use these approaches so well that eventually the parent's help should no longer be needed. The ultimate goal for all of these strategies is for your child to be able to trigger the "all clear" signal as needed to manage pain or stress.

A few tips before you get started:

◆ Practice the strategies in this section of the book yourself before trying to introduce them to your child. The confidence you gain from this step will make you a more effective teacher.

◆ When working with your child, set aside a short amount of time (ten to twenty minutes) when you won't be disrupted. Turn off cell phones, let siblings know you will be unavailable for those few minutes, and try to reduce outside noise.

◆ Introduce strategies at a time when your child is not in a pain flare or pain crisis. If these strategies are taught when your child has typical or low levels of pain, they can later be applied as needed when the pain is worse.

◆ Stick with it. It can take some practice to feel comfortable using these approaches, but it's worth it: many parents and kids I work with report that relaxation skills have become their go-to strategies for the management of pain.

10

A Better Breath

Many people have heard the advice "take a deep breath" when times are tough. This advice, while well intended, can seem overly simplistic and uncaring—as though the person suffering is somehow making a big deal out of nothing. But the simple fact is that learning structured deep-breathing strategies is probably the fastest, easiest, and most research-proven behavioral strategy to reduce pain and associated anxiety or stress. There are mountains of data and thousands of years of experience to back this up. New experimental research has even shown that deep, slow breathing in combination with relaxation is perhaps the most effective strategy a person can take to calm his or her autonomic nervous system. Moreover, deep breathing has been shown to slow the heart rate and relieve pain.

The diaphragm is a muscle that sits just below the rib cage, separating the lungs from the abdomen. The diaphragm's primary job is to control our respiration. When the diaphragm is at work, our belly gently rises and falls with each breath. You can clearly see this process when infants breathe and when most people are sleeping. The diaphragm, which naturally follows the arched contour of the ribs, flattens to pull air down through the lungs and into the abdomen with each inhalation, and arches up into a dome shape to push the air back out through the lungs with each exhalation. Because the abdomen, or belly, rises and falls with each diaphragmatic breath, this breathing technique is often called "belly breathing."

Many people wonder why it's necessary to teach children to use their diaphragm for breathing if the regulation of breathing is already the diaphragm's primary job. Why don't we just breathe like this all time? It's a good question. For reasons no one seems to understand, during the hustle and bustle of the day people often breathe more shallowly and bring air only into their lungs before exhaling. Poor posture or slouching, which compresses the diaphragm, may also limit diaphragmatic breathing during the day. Stress or pain can trigger more rapid and shallower breaths. And finally, people just get out of the habit of using their diaphragm for breathing during the day. Fortunately, it's fairly easy to restore the good habit of diaphragmatic breathing and take advantage of the benefits we get from letting the diaphragm do its work.

Diaphragmatic breathing has been proven to lower blood pressure, reduce stress, reduce pain, increase focus, improve concentration, and improve the function of the immune system. It's the most basic "do-it-anytime-and-anywhere" relaxation experience. Changing the way you breathe can make you feel relaxed, at ease, and more comfortable. Sometimes all it takes is four or five calming breaths to get back on track. But breathing in this smooth, rhythmic way for ten to fifteen minutes at a time will produce the best results.

Learning diaphragmatic breathing can be quick and easy. Getting kids to use it regularly can be a good bit trickier. I like to think that the process of getting kids to use this kind of breathing is similar to getting them to like a new food. If you have ever had a picky eater, you know that you need patience and persistence when introducing new foods. Many parents have heard the sage advice that getting a child to like a new food takes seven to nine exposures. In other words, a child might have to take "just one bite" of a green bean over seven to nine different meals in order to cultivate her acceptance or preference for green beans. For really picky eaters, it can take up to fifteen exposures.

This feeding advice is rooted in psychology research that finds that getting children used to new tastes and textures takes time and multiple experiences. Interestingly, this same body of research on eating new foods finds that parental attitudes about new foods are also very important. If parents show that they like green beans, eat green beans together with their children at mealtimes, and generally promote the tasting of new foods like green beans as a fun and enjoyable activity, kids are more likely to be accepting. Think about the introduction of diaphragmatic breathing as a new food. Model that you enjoy the breathing strategy, do it along with your child, and know that you may have to introduce the skill multiple times before your child accepts it as a worthwhile intervention. When children are first learning how to breathe this way they may find that it doesn't feel quite right or is hard to do, or they may rush to the conclusion that it doesn't lead to any benefit. Stick with it. Over time most children will report that diaphragmatic breathing feels natural and is a useful way to manage pain and pain-related stress.

Parents who learn diaphragmatic breathing gain another major advantage. When parents use this strategy it helps them to feel calm and relaxed, too—and this in turn can have a positive effect on their child's well-being. Research shows that when parents regulate their own heart rate and breathing they can more effectively respond to their child and move their child toward more adaptive coping. So even if your child won't fully participate at first, don't give up. The exercises may relax you and so in a very real way bring comfort to you both.

Over the past ten years I've had the good fortune of having a handful of the children and adolescents with whom I've worked come back to visit. I always ask if they are continuing to use their coping strategies and if so, which ones they use most. Without a doubt, diaphragmatic breathing is the most popular and enduring strategy of the bunch. Once kids learn how to make this technique work to their advantage, they seem to tuck the skill in their back pocket and pull it out whenever and wherever they need to relax.

Breathing in

As air passes through
the lungs, the diaphragm
moves downward to pull
the air into the belly (causing
the belly to expand).

Breathe in through the nose
for about 5 seconds

Diaphragm
contracts   Lung   Ribs

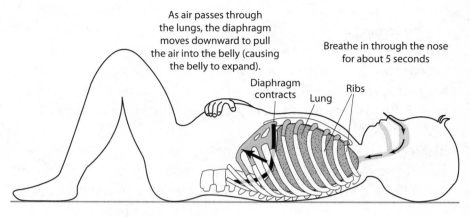

Breathing out

As air is exhaled,
the diaphragm relaxes,
helping to push air
out of the belly
and lungs.

Breathe out through the mouth
with lips pursed like you are
blowing through a straw
for about 5 seconds

Diaphragm
relaxes   Lung   Ribs

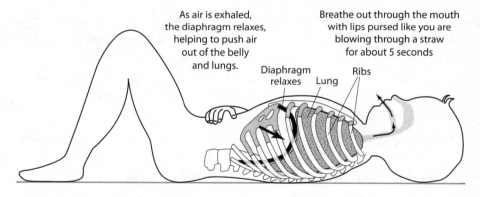

Diaphragmatic breathing.

How to Practice Diaphragmatic Breathing

◆ Lie down flat on your back with your knees bent, or sit up tall in a
chair. The most important part of the positioning is to ensure that
your abdomen is not crunched so that the diaphragm has plenty of
room to do its work.

◆ Place one hand on your abdomen, right over your belly button.
Place the other hand on your chest, right over your heart. Exhale all

of your air as slowly as possible. Imagine that you are blowing your air through a straw and can only release a bit at a time.

◆ As you release your air, feel your belly deflate, shoulders drop, and neck relax. Your joints and muscles will become loose and comfortable. Continue to deflate until you've released all the air from your belly and chest.

◆ When all your air is released, remain suspended in this quiet and peaceful state for a moment or two.

◆ When you're ready, slowly inhale your next breath in through your nose (as if you were smelling a flower) and into your lungs, filling your belly with air. Feel the hand on your chest rise as the air passes through your lungs and the hand on your belly rise as your diaphragm pulls the air down into your belly. You should feel your belly inflate like a balloon as you breathe in. Remember to keep your muscles calm and relaxed when you do this.

◆ Try breathing in for a count of five full seconds and then pausing for a moment. Pay attention to how still you can become when your mind is calm and focused only on your breath. Then slowly breathe out again, for a count of six to seven seconds. Exhale as if you were blowing through a straw, being sure to empty all the air in your belly and chest.

◆ Be patient with yourself. If you're not used to breathing in this way, it can take some practice until you feel at ease. Once you get a smooth, steady breath going, however, it should feel comfortable and relaxing to maintain this breathing pattern.

◆ Try to increase the number of breaths you can do in a row. Start with five breaths and try to work your way up to more. The ultimate goal might be ten or fifteen minutes of diaphragmatic breathing.

Variations

Spell it out. Sometimes it's fun to encourage children to do one breath for each letter in their first, middle, and last names. Alternatively they can spell out the names of a favorite singer or author, or spell the first names of their best friends.

Age up. Breathe one breath in and one breath out for each year your child is old counting up, and then one breath for each year counting back to zero. Try doing the ages of all siblings as well.

Buddy breathing. Sit face to face with your child and breathe together. If parents are practiced at diaphragmatic breathing, this can help to keep kids focused and on pace.

Mantra breathing. Have your child pick two words that have a special meaning or message and teach your child to say them silently in his or her mind with each breath. For example: "calm" (while breathing in) and "relaxed" (while breathing out). You can pick from the list below or have your child choose from his or her own favorite words.

- Peace . . . comfort
- Calm . . . breath
- I am . . . just fine
- I can . . . be well
- Cool . . . breeze
- Warm . . . sun
- More . . . at ease

Quick deflate. If you notice that your child is particularly tense or stressed or experiencing a high level of pain, have your child breathe out all of his or her air and imagine the whole body deflating like a balloon: the shoulders drop, arms relax, back softens, muscles release. Encourage your child to notice the difference between being tense and relaxed.

◆

How to Help

1. PICK THE RIGHT MOMENT TO START

Getting this breathing strategy down can take a bit of practice, especially for younger children, and it will be helpful overall if the first attempts are at least somewhat successful and pleasant. As with any new skill, it's hard to learn it when the pain or stress levels are high, so try to pick a time of day when your child is alert and calm.

2. TAKE IT SLOWLY

When you first introduce this skill, keep the practices very short, only one to two minutes. The diaphragm is a muscle and if your child is not used to breathing this way, it will fatigue quickly, making the skill harder to learn. However your child did, offer some meaningful praise and encouragement. Be positive. When you try again either later in the day or the next day, increase your practice time by only a minute or two.

3. PRACTICE WITH PROPS

Younger children or children with short attention spans often need visuals to keep their interest in this activity. You might:

◆ Place a small stuffed animal or favorite toy on your child's belly and see if your child can make the animal or toy rise and fall with each breath.
◆ Hold a pinwheel a few inches from your child's mouth so that with each slow breath out, your child can see his or her breath via the spinning of the pinwheel.
◆ Use bubbles as a way to engage a younger child. See how many bubbles your child can blow when exhaling.
◆ Give your child a party blower, harmonica, or whistle for an auditory cue when breathing out.
◆ Let your child place his or her hands on your belly to feel your rhythmic breathing. This can help to pace your child's breathing and serve as a relaxing way to connect around this useful strategy.

4. DON'T FOCUS ON THE PAIN

Most children do find that this breathing strategy reduces pain and increases feelings of relaxation. In the beginning, however, it's helpful to focus more on the process of learning the technique and engaging in the strategy and less on the outcomes. So don't ask your child if he or she feels better afterward. If your child comments that it was or wasn't helpful, simply acknowledge the comment.

5. FOCUS ON A STEADY BREATH

Traditionally, diaphragmatic breaths are made up of a five-second inhale and five-second exhale. But this is just a general guideline. Some people find that they can only breathe in for four seconds, but can breathe out for eight seconds. It's completely fine to allow your child to find his or her own ideal breath count. The focus should be on establishing a smooth, slow, rhythmic breath where the inhalation corresponds to an inflated belly and the exhalation corresponds to a flattened belly.

6. KEEP IT COMFORTABLE

For some children, especially those with abdominal pain, a fully inflated belly breath can feel painful. If this is the case, suggest that your child breathe in less air, stopping the inhale before it reaches a point of discomfort. If your child can inhale for only one to two seconds, that's fine. Just hold that breath and exhale as slowly as possible (probably six to seven seconds). Again, the goal is to obtain a slow, steady, rhythmic breath. The size of the breath is less important.

7. USE TECHNOLOGY TO HONE YOUR SKILLS

If this technique is new to you, Google "diaphragmatic breathing" and you will find several useful video clips that demonstrate this technique. There are also many smartphone apps currently available that help to reinforce diaphragmatic breathing (see Appendix 3). These apps can help kids to establish and maintain a slow steady breath, provide an incentive for slowly increasing the length of practice, and serve as an engaging visual or auditory aid that can help children stay focused on the skill.

11
Connecting Mind to Body through Story

Stories are not just frivolous tales for little kids. We learn much about the world we live in through stories. In fact, some experts argue that our evolution has depended in part on the human brain's ability to assimilate new information by creating and sharing stories. Imagine for a moment what it would be like if you had to experience everything in the world first-hand. Our fund of knowledge would be so small that we'd struggle to make any real progress in our world. For example, most people don't hitchhike because it can be an unsafe practice. How do we know this? Clearly not everyone has hitchhiked before and had a bad experience. But most everyone has heard a version of a story about a hitchhiker who never made it to his or her destination. If the story is really compelling, many people will have a physical reaction to the story such as having "chills" or the feeling of the little hairs on the back of one's neck standing on end. That reaction is the brain responding as if the situation was a real threat, not just a story.

Over the past ten years a new wave of research using positron emission tomography (PET) and functional magnetic resonance imaging (fMRI) has shown that mental imagery can trigger the same neurobiological activity as actual perception. This means that mental imagery and real life experiences can both elicit responses from the same memory, emotion, and motor-control centers in the brain. For example, listening to a scary story while in an fMRI scanner can show activation in the amygdala, a key area of the brain that regulates the fight or flight response. It's thought that our brain's capacity to respond to stories with mind and body may have evolved as part of our evolutionary protection plan, and we can harness this power to our advantage.

Guided imagery is a technique that capitalizes on the fact that stories have the power to make our brain work "as if." Guided imagery feeds your brain sensory-rich information and your body responds as if this information is real. So while you may not be able to leave tonight on a plane to Hawaii, if you hear a story that vividly details a lazy stroll along the shimmering sands of a Hawaiian cove, you can trick your brain into triggering the type of relaxation response you might experience if you were actually there.

Here I will review the basic tenets of how to engage your child with guided imagery, using multiple examples and specific scripts. Parents can read the scripts directly to their child, or modify them to meet their child's individual needs.

How to Trigger the "as if" Effect

Some of the best guided-imagery stories for helping to relax and distract children may vary from what is typically thought of as "relaxing." Kids have the unique and wonderful ability to use their imaginations to help them feel better. The key is to think about what your child truly loves and to integrate that into a sensory-rich story. In the past I've created *Star Wars*–themed guided-imagery stories, dance recital stories, cliff diving stories, deep sea fishing stories, roller coaster stories, and farming stories, just to name a few. Sometimes kids have to try a variety of guided-imagery stories before they get the hang of it and want to help create or modify their own story. Other times, kids know right from the start that they want to go to a particular favorite place and have many ideas for how to create the "as if" experience. As a general rule, younger children may have better attention for action-packed stories like playing baseball on a warm summer day or swimming like a fish through cool waters, while adolescents may prefer more passive stories such as the imagined experience of being stretched out on a soft sandy beach or wandering slowly down a wooded path.

One of the most helpful strategies for creating a good "as if" guided-imagery story is to include details that supply information to all five senses: a really engaging story will include descriptive information for sight, sound, smell, taste, and feel. For example, when creating a guided-imagery story about a trip to an amusement park, you can include phrases like "*see* the many rides including the roller coaster, spinning tea cups, and rocking pirate ship; *hear* the lively sounds of the music and the sound of kids laughing and screaming on the rides; *smell* the yummy burgers and hot dogs on the grill and the sweet scent of freshly spun cotton candy; *taste* a cool slushy followed by a bite of salty popcorn; *feel* the warm summer sun on the top of your head and shoulders and the wind in your hair as you run full speed toward your favorite ride." Details like these will captivate your child. There are truly an infinite number of possibilities for creating guided-imagery stories for your child. Children may enjoy the challenge of trying new stories each time they practice guided imagery, or they might find one or two stories that they really enjoy and want to return to again and again.

Plan to spend about eight to fifteen minutes on a guided-imagery story. First invite your child to close his eyes. Next have your child focus on his breath and on releasing tension in the body and mind by leading him through some diaphragmatic breathing cycles and by making suggestions about settling comfortably into the chair or bed or wherever your child may be. Tell the guided-imagery story in a slow, soft, calm voice. The slow pacing is particularly important because it gives your child's brain time to more deeply process the information; this creates a stronger image and generates emotional links to the story. It can be helpful to pause briefly between segments of the story, and these pauses can increase in length as your child becomes more deeply relaxed.

As you're telling a story, make *suggestions* for what your child may experience, but allow some room for your child to actively engage his own imagination. For example, if you are continuing the earlier story about an amusement park, instead of suggesting "Enjoy a sip of a cool blue-raspberry slushy," you could say, "Now imagine that your cup is filled with your favorite slushy flavor. It could be strawberry, fruit punch, blue raspberry, lemonade, cola, or any other flavor. Whatever you choose." Inviting this level of participation will further engage your child. Sometimes children like to talk while they are participating in a guided-imagery story. For example, some kids might want to share, "I picked a lemonade slushy!" This is perfectly fine. You can simply acknowledge the choice and keep going. Alternatively, you can ask your child to describe what the slushy tastes like and this can help to deepen the experience of relaxation. While your child is engaged in the story, it can be helpful to cue your child to take a deep breath. For example, in the amusement park story you can say, "Take a nice deep breath and enjoy the scent of the sweet cotton candy, then breathe out slowly and relax."

Using Guided Imagery to Ease Pain

Beyond creating general feelings of relaxation, the power of story and suggestion can also be used to change physical sensations. Ever notice how just *thinking* about fingernails running down a chalkboard can create the physical sensation of chills running down your spine? That same type of mind-body connection can be used to trick the brain into modifying physical sensations that might be associated with pain or discomfort.

Guided imagery can alter the sensation of pain in a number of ways. One type of guided-imagery story can change pain by offering a child a new paradigm for thinking about his or her pain. These stories may make suggestions about how big the pain is, how much control the child has over the pain, and the amount of worry or distress the child needs to feel about the pain. When children are given a new paradigm or construct for thinking about pain within a guided imagery, they may then be able to alter the amount of distress they feel. These changes can happen quickly and can in some cases have a lasting effect on a child's experience of pain.

There are also types of guided-imagery stories that are designed specifically to target physiological sensation. These are often referred to as "autogenic relaxation" stories. Autogenic means self-generated. This type of guided-imagery story involves making suggestions about how to change one's sensory experience, and it can be used to transform pain or discomfort into more pleasant sensations. Keep in mind that it's best to personalize autogenic relaxation stories to fit your child's specific discomfort. So if your child has burning, hot pain, the autogenic suggestion could be a cooling sensation; if your child has headaches, autogenic suggestions for warm hands and feet have been shown to reduce headache pain; and if your child has sharp pain, autogenic suggestions for a gentle tingling sensation may be comforting. Many autogenic relaxation stories are designed to promote feeling warm, heavy, and relaxed since these sensations are frequently effective for reducing pain and often help people to feel more relaxed in general. Before using such a story, though, parents should be sure to check with their child to see if "warm and heavy" are sensory experiences that will bring their child comfort. If not, they can simply exchange those words with others that their child feels will be more helpful, like "cool and calm" or "gentle tingle."

Some Guided-Imagery Stories to Try

Truly any story can be an "as if" guided-imagery story. What's most important is making sure a child is connected to his or her story. This means that having a child's input and allowing a child to modify the story is an important part of the process. For example, I once suggested to a seven-year-old boy that we try a guided-imagery story where we imagined painting a soothing color over the areas of his body where he was tense. I suggested that the special paint would relax his body and change his sensation of discomfort. I called it a "paint story." We practiced it a few times and then he said, "Let's call it 'zaint' instead of paint, and let's have the 'zaint' absorb into the top of my head, sink into my brain, wash out my worry thoughts and make my whole body feel calm and peaceful." So that's what we did. Not surprisingly, because he had an active role in creating the guided imagery, the "zaint" worked beautifully to reduce his stress and pain. We practiced "zaint" regularly and he eventually learned to do "zaint" on his own with the simple tactile trigger of just touching the top of his head.

I happen to think that parents are naturally wonderful at coming up with engaging guided-imagery stories for their kids. But if you prefer to use a script, reading guided-imagery stories can be equally as effective. Here are examples of scripts you can try with your child. Each has a "stay awake" ending and a "go to sleep" ending. Because guided-imagery stories can be very useful for helping children to fall asleep, many parents use these stories at bedtime. But guided imagery can also provide a much needed break during the day, especially when your child is feeling a lot of stress or pain. If you are using these scripts during the day, read the "stay awake" ending. If you are using these scripts before bedtime, select the "go to sleep" ending.

SCRIPT FOR PAIN REDUCTION (ALL AGES)

Let's start by taking a few slow, deep breaths. Breathe in through your nose and out through your mouth. Just pace yourself in a way that feels comfortable, smooth, and easy. Breathe in through your nose, pulling the air down into your belly, pause for just a moment, then breathe your air out through your mouth. With each breath in, you are becoming more and more relaxed. With each breath out, you are feeling calm and comfortable. Slow and steady. Release any tension. Relax now and give your body time to heal. Relax now and know that this is just what you are supposed to do. Now that your breath is slow and steady, and you've begun to relax, we're going to use the power of your mind to change your sensation of pain. It will be interesting to see in what ways this will change your experience of pain today.

Close your eyes. This will help your imagination to do its best work. Now imagine the color of your pain. Perhaps it is bright red like a fire. It might be a dull, dark color like steel gray. Perhaps it is icy blue.

Once you can clearly see the color of your pain, think about the shape of your pain. Is it a round blob? Does it have sharp pointy edges? Does it look like a familiar object? Take a moment to think about the shape of your pain.

Now that you see the color and the shape, think about the size. Is your pain small and just in the area where it hurts you most? Is your pain large and taking over your body? Think about how big this pain is.

Now that you have a clear picture of the color, shape, and size of your pain, we're ready to take a trip to the central control station in your brain. To do this, use your eyes to look inward. Watch as you navigate through your brain. Up and down all of the structures in your mind. Traveling deep into your brain, you are looking for a control board. Your control board will be a panel with a lot of levers and dials. This control panel is responsible for the color, shape, and size of your pain. Take your time to reach the control center. Once you're there, take three slow deep breaths (pause while your child breathes).

Now your task is to find the lever to change the size of your pain. The lever is marked with zero at the bottom and ten at the top. Pulling this lever will change the size of your pain. This is actually a very heavy lever, but you find when you reach up to grab it that you are stronger than you thought. You reach up to this large lever and begin to pull. Notice as you take the lever from ten down to eight that the size of your pain has begun to shrink. Apply pressure to this lever and shrink your pain from an eight to a six. Continue to pull on this lever and keep watching as your pain continues to shrink, from a six to a four, and now from a four to a two. And now pull it all the way down to the bottom and notice how small the size of your pain has become.

Now that you've got this smaller, much more manageable piece of pain, I want you to look in your control center for a color dial. This dial shows the color of your pain. So if you identified your pain as being red, this dial is red. If your pain was gray, or blue, or purple, the dial will also be that color. Find the dial on the control panel. Once you're there, take three slow deep breaths (pause while your child breathes).

If you look closely at this color dial, you'll see around the dial there is a color guide that goes from a bright color to a very pale color. For example, it might go from bright red to pale pink, or from dark blue to a light sky blue. Your job now is to turn the dial from the intense color to the palest color. Turn it slowly and carefully and watch as your piece of pain transforms from being intensely colored to being very pale. It may even appear transparent or completely see-through. Take your time. It's sometimes very easy to turn this dial, and sometimes it takes a little bit of effort. When you've reached the palest, lightest, most-see-through color on your dial, take three nice, slow, deep breaths (pause while your child breathes).

Now all we have left to do is to transform the shape of this piece of pain. You've now got a small, softly colored piece of pain. The last step is the easiest. This requires very little effort. Look on your control panel for a touch screen. You'll see the shape of your pain on this touch screen panel. You can now gently touch any sharp edges on your piece of pain. When you touch these edges on the touch screen, they will become soft and smooth. You can also drag lines on this touchscreen to change the shape entirely. Now is your opportunity to change your pain into a soft, flexible shape without any hard edges. Make it smooth. Make it soft. When you're done, take three slow, deep, relaxing breaths (pause while your child breathes).

Very nicely done. Now, with your eyes still closed, take a moment to see what your pain looks like. Notice how much smaller, lighter, softer, and more transparent your pain has become. You may have even been so successful that your pain has become too small to see. If so, that's wonderful!

Take a moment to really enjoy this experience. Be aware of how still your arms and legs have become. Perhaps your body feels heavier or warmer than before. With every slow deep breath, notice how peaceful your body feels.

Stay Awake Ending

I'm going to count down from ten slowly and when I reach one, you can open your eyes. Know that you can carry this relaxing and comfortable feeling with you even after you open your eyes. This feeling is yours to enjoy.

10 . . . 9 . . . 8 . . . Become aware of the room around you

7 . . . 6 . . . 5 . . . Take a deep breath and start to wiggle your fingers and toes

4 . . . 3 . . . 2 . . . Give a big head to toe stretch

1 . . . Open your eyes, feeling calm and refreshed.

Go to Sleep Ending

I'm going to slowly count down from ten and when I reach one, you can peacefully drift off into a deep and comfortable sleep.

10 . . . 9 . . . 8 . . . Feeling calm and relaxed

7 . . . 6 . . . 5 . . . Easing into sleep

4 . . . 3 . . . 2 . . . More and more relaxed

1 . . . Drifting comfortably to sleep.

SCRIPT FOR GENERAL RELAXATION (ALL AGES)

Take a few slow, deep breaths to get started. Breathe in through your nose and out through your mouth. Pace yourself in a way that feels comfortable, smooth, and easy. Breathe in through your nose, pulling the air down into your belly, pause for just a moment, then breathe your air out through your mouth. With each breath in, you are becoming more and more relaxed. With each breath out, you are feeling calm and comfortable. Slow and steady. Release any tension. Relax now giving your body time to heal. Relax now and know that this is just what you are supposed to do.

Now turn your attention to your right hand. Feel the skin on the palm of your right hand becoming soft and relaxed. Feel the sensation of warmth and comfort spread to each finger, to the back of your hand, to your wrist, and your entire arm.

Your right arm is starting to feel very heavy. Very heavy, and very relaxed. Your right arm is heavy, warm, and relaxed.

Now focus on your left hand. Feel your left hand relaxing completely. Allow your wrist to soften and relax. Your left arm is becoming heavy and warm. Allow your left arm to sink into comfort. Your left arm feels heavy, warm, and relaxed.

Now turn your attention to your legs. Feel your legs becoming calm and relaxed. Feel the sensation of warmth, heaviness, and comfort spreading all the way from your feet to your ankles to your lower legs, knees, and hips. Feel your legs becoming heavy. Very warm, heavy, and very relaxed. Your legs are warm, heavy, and relaxed.

Imagine a warm, gentle breeze blowing across your face. Feel your forehead, cheeks, chin, and lips becoming soft and relaxed. Feel the heaviness of your eyelids and allow them to relax as well.

Now imagine a soothing sun shining down on you and relaxing the whole front of your body. Allow your chest and stomach to relax. Your entire front of your body feels warm and heavy. Feel the sun shining and warming your skin. Relax more and more as the whole front of your body is filled with warmth and calm, pleasant relaxation.

Now imagine the soothing sun shining on your back. Feel your back getting warm, heavy, and relaxed. Notice how the feelings of warmth and relaxation spread all the way from your neck to your shoulders to your upper back, middle back, and lower back. Feel your whole back relaxing as it becomes warm, heavy, and relaxed. Feel the heaviness in your entire body. Your body from your head to your toes is warm, heavy, calm, and relaxed.

Enjoy this calm, relaxed feeling. Notice your smooth, even breathing. Each deep breath draws you even further into relaxation. Your body feels very warm, heavy, calm, relaxed, and comfortable. Enjoy the relaxation for a few more moments (pause for a minute or two).

Stay Awake Ending

Now slowly begin to bring your attention back to this room. Keeping your eyes closed, bring your awareness to the surface that you are resting on, hear the sounds in your environment, gently start to reawaken your body. Wiggle your fingers and toes, move your arms and legs a little, and give a head-to-toe stretch if you would like to do so. Whenever you are ready, you can open your eyes and become fully alert.

Go to Sleep Ending

I'm going to count down from ten slowly and when I reach one, you can peacefully drift off into a deep and comfortable sleep.
10 . . . 9 . . . 8 . . . Feeling calm and relaxed
7 . . . 6 . . . 5 . . . Easing gently into sleep
4 . . . 3 . . . 2 . . . More and more relaxed
1 . . . Resting comfortably as you drift off to sleep.

SCRIPT FOR GENERAL RELAXATION (AGES 6–11)

Let's start by breathing deeply and relaxing your whole body from your head to your toes. First empty out all of your air with a big exhale. Ahhhh. Now breathe in through your nose and fill your belly with fresh air. When you are ready, breathe out slowly just like you are breathing out through a straw. Slow and steady. Easy and calm. With each breath in, you become more and more relaxed. With each breath out, you feel more calm and comfortable. Slow and steady. Release any tension. Settle in now; become more and more relaxed. Set aside any worries or concerns. Know that right now, at this moment, your only job is just to relax. Relax now and give your body time to heal. Feel the pleasant sensation of relaxation spread from the very top of your head, over your eyes, across your face, down your neck, across your shoulders, down your arms, through each fingertip, to your chest and belly, easing your breath more and more. Feel the relaxation through your hips, spreading down your legs all the way through your toes. Take a deep breath in and enjoy these sensations of relaxation. Breathe out slowly, clearing your mind completely.

Now, allow your eyes to close and imagine you are going for a walk in big grassy field. The grass is bright green and the sky above is a clear blue. Kick off your shoes and socks and feel the cool blades of grass between your toes. Begin to make your way into the center of the field and as you get close to the center, notice that there is a small red airplane resting in the middle of the field. As you get closer and closer, you realize that this is a glider plane and that it's just your size. It's got a single seat, long graceful wings, and a small engine. Make your way over to the airplane, climb inside the open cockpit, and fasten your seatbelt. Once you are comfortable inside, look along the front of the plane until you find a red start button. Push the button and listen as the small engine begins to hum. Hummmm. Can you hear it? Good. Feel the gentle vibrations in the plane as the engine hums a little bit louder, signaling that the plane is ready to go. Now the plane begins to roll through the field and you are filled with feelings of calm and joy as you prepare for your journey. The plane rolls faster and faster and you feel safe and well supported in your seat. Feel the gentle liftoff as the plane takes flight and notice how free and weightless you feel in the air. Feel the gentle sway of the plane in the sky, softly soaring, so peaceful and calm.

Once in the sky, your humming engine becomes quiet and you glide effortlessly through the air. You are in complete control of your plane. You can choose to go fast or slow. You can choose to go way up high into the clouds or stay low near the ground. You steer your plane simply by thinking about where you would like it to go. Think the word "up" if you want to go up. Or think the word "down" if you'd like the plane to go down. If you see something interesting, just think about whatever it is and the plane will take you there.

While in the air, your only job is to collect memories of the beautiful things that you see, feel, and touch. You can do this by paying very close attention to the things around you. Start by paying attention to the clouds in the sky. What shapes do you see? Are the clouds thick and fluffy? Or soft and wispy? Are there many clouds throughout the sky or just a few?

Now notice the trees around you. Glide slowly so you can pay close attention to all the different kinds of trees you see. Can you see trees with apples or pears? Do you see pine trees with pinecones? Can you find tall skinny trees? Or trees with really thick trunks? While you're looking at the trees notice any birds' nests tucked into the branches. Perhaps you can even find a mother or father bird feeding the babies, or helping to build the nest.

Listen to the sounds that you hear on your special plane ride. First notice the sound of the air as you soar through the sky. Now listen to other sounds you might hear. Do you hear birds chirping or sing-ing? Can you hear the bubbling water of a nearby river? Perhaps you can hear the rustling of leaves in the trees. Listen carefully to the sounds.

Now pay close attention to the weather around you. Do you feel warm and relaxed on a bright summer day? Or are you enjoying the sensation of a cool and breezy autumn day? Is it damp and dewy on your skin? Or is your skin warm and dry?

Last but not least, pay close attention to how you are feeling on this plane ride. This is part of your memory, too. As you breathe deeply, pay attention to your body and mind. Notice how the muscles in your body have become soft, relaxed, comfortable, and at ease. Notice that your mind may feel lighter, less worried, and more calm. Pay attention to the positive feelings that you may have. Notice feelings of happiness, contentment, joy, or gratitude. Whatever your feelings may be.

Now that you've collected all of these memories from your trip, in-cluding the sights, sounds, and feelings, your job is to tuck these memo-ries into a part of your mind that will keep them safe and protected. Take a moment to tuck these away. Perhaps there is a special box or envelope in your mind or just a special part of your brain that will hold these memories. Wherever you decide to leave them, just remember where they are so you can come back to them anytime you wish.

With your memories stored safely in your mind, your plane slowly begins to make its safe and easy descent back into the grassy green field. Watch comfortably as you get closer to the ground, rocking gently side to side. A gentle bounce signals that you're on the ground and rolling across the field. You can feel the ground beneath the wheels of the plane as your plane slows and finally comes to a stop. Unfasten your seatbelt and climb out of the cockpit, once again feeling the cool grass between your toes and on the bottoms of your feet and once again smelling the fresh clean air. Slowly make your way back to the edge of the field where your shoes and socks are waiting for you. As you make your way back across the field notice that you continue to feel light and airy, relaxed and comfortable. Notice that things that may have been bothering you earlier now seem to bother you very little if at all. Take a deep breath in and enjoy this feeling of satisfaction and comfort.

Stay Awake Ending

Before ending your trip, check to be sure the memories from your plane ride are tucked safely in your mind. Know that you can go back to those memories and feelings anytime you wish. Now take a deep breath in and when you breathe out wiggle your fingers and toes. Take another deep breath in and when you breathe this time, stretch your arms and legs. Take one more deep breath in, and this time, when you exhale, open your eyes feeling awake and refreshed.

Go to Sleep Ending

Your plane ride has helped you feel so relaxed and at ease. Falling asleep now will be easy and fast. Allow the special memories that you collected to fill your dreams, providing feelings of comfort and peace all through the night.

SCRIPT FOR GENERAL RELAXATION (AGES 12 AND UP)

Take a deep breath in and when you breathe out, relax your whole body from your head to your toes. Now take three slow, steady breaths. Find your own pace. Breathe in through your nose, pulling the air down into your belly, pausing for just a moment, then breathe your air out through your mouth. Slow and steady. Easy and effortless. With each breath in, you are becoming more and more relaxed. With each breath out, you are feeling calm and comfortable. Slow and steady. Release any tension. Settle in now and become more and more relaxed. Any worries or concerns are just set aside. Feel the sensation of relaxation spread from the very top of your head, over your eyes, across your face, down your neck, across your shoulders, down your arms, through each fingertip, to your chest and belly—easing your breath more and more. Feel the relaxation through your hips, spreading down your thighs, knees, calves, feet, and all the way through your toes. Take a deep breath in and enjoy these sensations of relaxation. Breathe out slowly, clearing your mind completely.

Now that you are feeling relaxed and at ease, close your eyes and imagine that stretched out in front of you, as far as you can see, is a glistening white sand beach with aqua blue waters hugging the shore. This private beach is yours to enjoy. It's a beautiful summer day and the sun is directly above, shining down on the top of your head, the back of your neck, your shoulders, arms, legs, and the tops of your feet. Now you begin walking down the beach, feeling the powder-soft sand under the arch of your foot and through your toes. Listen closely to the sounds you hear on this peaceful beach. You hear the soft rhythmic crashing of the waves against the sandy shore, the distant sound of seagulls, and the windlike rustling of sails from a faraway sailboat. These gentle sounds relax you more and more, helping you to feel peaceful and at ease, calm and relaxed. Take in a deep breath of fresh, salty sea air. Breathe the air deeply into your belly and, as you exhale, notice the taste of the salty sea air on your lips.

As you make your way down the beach, feel the cool, relaxing sensation of a gentle breeze across your face and shoulders. It's blowing gently and softly, cooling your warm skin. Up ahead in the distance, you see a smooth rock face jutting out into the clear blue ocean. Make your way over to this rock face and climb up to the top. Notice all of the smooth contours of the rock and walk across this smooth rock surface until you find the contours that fit your body perfectly. Stretch out on the warm rock so that your arms and legs are completely extended. Notice how your chest opens up and your breathing becomes truly effortless. Enjoy the warmth of the rock, the sun, and the gentle ocean breeze. As you breathe in a deep breath, pay attention to your body and mind. Notice that the muscles in your body are soft, relaxed, comfortable, and at ease. Notice that your mind may feel lighter, have less worry, or be calmer. Pay attention to positive feelings that may have arisen. While stretched out on this rock you may feel happy, content, joyful, or grateful. Whatever your feelings may be, for the next minute just relax and enjoy these feelings and the sights, sounds, and sensations you have noticed on the beach. At the end of one minute you will hear my voice again. (Wait one minute.)

Stay Awake Ending

Now that you are completely relaxed, you are ready to make your way back from the beach. Slowly roll over on the rock so that you can easily push yourself to a sitting position. Now stand up and stretch your arms into the warmth of the sun. Begin to walk down the beach back to your starting point. As you near your starting point, take a deep breath in and when you breathe out, gently wiggle your fingers and toes. Take another deep breath in and when you breathe out this time, stretch your arms and legs. When you finally reach your starting point, take one more deep breath in and when you exhale, open your eyes feeling awake and refreshed.

Go to Sleep Ending

Resting peacefully on this rock is the perfect place to drift off into a deep and comfortable sleep. Notice how fully supported you feel by the contours of the warm rock. Notice how safe and peaceful you feel on this quiet, private beach. I will count to five and when I reach five you can fall into a deep, comfortable, and peaceful sleep.

1 . . . Feeling more and more relaxed

2 . . . Deeper and deeper into relaxation

3 . . . Feeling calm and at ease

4 . . . More and more relaxed

5 . . . Drifting softly and effortlessly into sleep.

More Guided-Imagery Story Ideas

You may embellish the following story ideas to extend them into longer, full-length stories. Or you can simply share these ideas with your child and let him or her create a comforting and relaxing experience. Encourage your child to close his or her eyes and try to create an engaging story independently.

- Experience a ski slope on a cool but sunny winter day. Feel the cool breeze on your face as you swoosh down the slope, listen to your skis as they race through the snow, take a deep breath of the fresh mountain air, and enjoy the majestic mountain views.

- Imagine you are in your room wearing your most comfortable pajamas. Taste the cool, fresh toothpaste on your just-brushed teeth, then snuggle into your bed and enjoy the "just right" feeling of your soft sheets, your fluffy pillow, and the perfect weight of your blanket. Hear your favorite music playing faintly in the background, smell the cool clean night air, and drift off to sleep.

- Pretend you are on a soccer field in the final seconds of the game and it's your turn with the ball. Run down the field while you feel the wind blow in your hair, the sweat drip down your face, and the sun shine on the top of your head. Inhale the fresh scent of the freshly mowed field. Focus on the goal, shoot, and score!

- It's a baseball game with the bases loaded in the bottom of the ninth. At your next up at bat, listen to the crowd roar, see the narrowing of the pitcher's eyes, feel the whoosh of the fast ball headed your way, watch in slow motion as you swing the bat, hear the loud "crack" when the bat makes contact with the ball, and watch as it soars through the clear blue sky . . . going, going, gone! It's a grand slam! Run the bases and bask in the cheers of the crowd!

◆ You are walking through a forest surrounded by tall pine trees. Listen for a bubbling brook, smell the wet leaves on the ground, relax on a cool moss-covered rock, and feel a gentle rain shower on your skin.

◆

How to Help

1. TALK WITH YOUR CHILD ABOUT THE POWER OF STORIES

Let your child know that stories can make our mind and body feel "as if" we are really experiencing the situation being described. Guided-imagery exercises are designed to help relax our mind and body, creating feelings of comfort and calm.

2. SET ASIDE SOME QUIET TIME

Turn off cell phones and find a time during the day when you and your child will not be interrupted for at least fifteen minutes. Bedtime can be the perfect time to try guided-imagery exercises.

3. FIRST TRY IT WHEN THE PAIN IS NOT SEVERE

Avoid first practicing a new relaxation skill like guided imagery when your child is at his or her worst; instead try it out when the situation is more stable. Once your child has had some experience with guided imagery, it will be an excellent strategy to use during episodes of increased pain.

4. HELP YOUR CHILD TO DEVELOP A PERSONAL RELAXATION SCRIPT

You can discuss the types of things your child finds interesting or relaxing. Sometimes it's helpful to try out a promising script, then adjust it to make the story feel "just right."

5. DIVE IN

One of the most common statements I hear from parents is that they feel they "just don't know how to do this right." Truly there is not a wrong way. If a particular script or story doesn't work for your child, simply make adjustments and try again. Keep the lines of communication open with your child. Would they prefer that you talk faster? Softer? Include a favorite pet? Leave out parts of the story? Whatever makes your child feel the most comfortable is the way to go. If your child would prefer to practice guided imagery independently, feel free to try some of the apps I recommend in Appendix 3.

6. PROCESS THE EXPERIENCE

After completing a guided-imagery exercise, give your child a little time to revive completely then ask your child what the experience was like. Can he recall images or feelings? Which ones? Don't focus on whether the story reduced pain, but do draw your child's attention to the positive sensations and emotions that emerged. If your child felt relaxed and comfortable, you will know that this was a helpful experience. If your child didn't feel good about the process, talk about what got in the way and try again another time with a different script.

7. RECORD YOUR PRACTICE

Reading or telling a guided-imagery story can be a wonderfully supportive way to connect with a child. But parents aren't always around and sometimes adolescents prefer to be more independent while relaxing. One way to get around these challenges is to use a trick that therapists frequently use to encourage home-based practice. Simply use the memo feature in your child's favorite smartphone or tablet device and record your practice as a memo. Then your child can listen to you tell the guided-imagery story any time of day or night.

12

Targeting Muscle Tension

When a person experiences pain, the body automatically tries to protect the painful area by tightening the muscles nearby. This part of our body's defense system contributes to the cycle of pain, because tense muscles themselves can lead to pain. For children with persistent pain, the muscles around the area with pain are often chronically tight. Muscles that aren't even near the area of discomfort can become tense, which also exacerbates pain. For example, children with abdominal pain may frequently hunch over, holding their bellies in discomfort, which sometimes leads to back and neck pain.

Muscle pain and tension can also result from inactivity. Our bodies are meant for movement, and when children are less active either as a result of pain or illness or because they prefer more sedentary activities (such as watching TV or playing on the computer), muscles, tendons, and ligaments begin to lose their flexibility. As a result, children can develop muscle imbalances, with some muscles staying too tightly contracted and others becoming too weak to contract properly. Children with chronic pain may also at times have muscle tension from bursts of overactivity. While activity is generally a good idea for children, sometimes a sudden increase in activity after a long break can cause temporary soreness or muscle tension.

Stress and anxiety are also primary causes of muscle tension. When we feel anxious or stressed, our muscles become more rigid. This muscle rigidity happens without any conscious effort and is related to our body's fight or flight defense. When we are chronically in a state of stress or anxiety, our muscles are primed for action at any time. Being in a constant state of readiness is tough work for the muscles; they respond to the persistent call for action with muscle fatigue and pain. They can also respond with muscle cramping and spasm. In fact, persistent muscle tension or a muscle spasm—especially in the neck, back, or jaw—is one of the hallmark signs of anxiety and is often reported to doctors before chronic anxiety or stress is even recognized as a problem.

For all of these reasons, finding strategies to relieve and reduce muscle tightness and tension is very important. We all have occasionally felt stiff muscles upon waking in the morning or after a strenuous day of exercise. Usually a few good stretches combined with the normal activity of starting the day helps to lessen these mild muscle tensions. When you stretch or start moving in your day, your brain sends much needed blood and oxygen to these muscles, helping them to slowly release, reducing soreness and facilitating an ease of movement. When a person is in pain and is actively guarding against using her muscles, is unable to get out of bed and get moving with the day, or has persistent tightness due to muscle overuse, these muscles may not have the opportunity to release and relax. Muscle relaxation strategies are designed to reduce the discomfort associated with muscle tension and musculoskeletal pain. They help teach the body how to relax even when pain or stress is present and importantly teach the mind to be aware of the difference between tense and relaxed muscles. These muscle relaxation strategies can also generate more widespread feelings of calm and relaxation.

Most muscle relaxation techniques are termed "progressive muscle relaxation." This means that muscle tension is targeted in a progressive fashion, either from the head to the toes, or toes to the head. This progression helps to create a wave of muscle relaxation that feels as if it's slowly washing up or down the body. It also helps to bring a person's attention to the difference between tense and relaxed muscles in a programmatic way. After all, it's far easier (and more effective) to focus on one small group of muscles at a time rather than all the muscles all at once.

Progressive muscle relaxation can actually be done in one of two ways. One can either actively tense then release each muscle group in the body, or one can simply focus on releasing tension (without tensing the muscle first). Purposefully tensing each muscle group brings blood and oxygen to the muscle and surrounding tissues and this helps to further relax the muscle group, but some people prefer to skip the tensing and just focus on the relaxing part of the experience.

Similar to guided-imagery stories, muscle relaxation techniques are very helpful for reducing stress, easing pain, alleviating anxiety, promoting feelings of wellness, and improving sleep. One recent study even found that progressive muscle relaxation was equivalent to the powerful anxiolytic (anti-anxiety medication) Diazepam in terms of both a person's subjective experience of relaxation and the physiological biomarkers for stress (blood glucose levels).

How to Progressively Relax Your Muscles

Progressive muscle relaxation is best done lying down on a bed or stretched out on the floor, but it can also be done in a chair if needed. Similar to a guided-imagery story, parents can read one of the scripts below or generate a script for their child based on his or her particular needs. It's helpful to have a child use diaphragmatic breathing throughout a progressive muscle relaxation exercise. It's also helpful to cue a child when to take a deep breath during a progressive muscle relaxation exercise since many children are prone to hold their breath when they tense their muscles. As a general guideline, you can suggest that your child hold each muscle group tight for ten to fifteen seconds, then let the muscles relax for five to ten seconds. Relaxation in each muscle group can be enhanced by repeating the tense-and-release cycle so that the muscles are tensed and relaxed twice before moving on to the next area. The first time a muscle is tightened and then released, the muscle is primed. This priming seems to enhance the feelings of relaxation during the second muscle tense-and-release cycle. It's important to let your child know that he or she should hold the muscle as tight as possible without straining. If your child anticipates that tensing a particular muscle will be too uncomfortable, simply have your child imagine tensing the muscle. The effect can be similar.

SCRIPT FOR ACTIVE PROGRESSIVE MUSCLE RELAXATION

Take a few slow, deep breaths to get started. Breathe in through your nose and out through your mouth. Pace yourself in a way that feels comfortable, smooth, and easy. Breathe in through your nose, pulling the air down into your belly, pause for just a moment, then breathe your air out through your mouth. With each breath in, you are becoming more and more relaxed. As you breathe out, imagine that the tension in your body is draining away. Find the pace that is right for you. Easy, effortless, and relaxed. Slow and steady. Release any tension.

Now, in order to get your muscles to relax, we're going to tighten each muscle group for about ten seconds and then allow each muscle group to relax for about ten seconds. Try to keep your attention focused on each muscle group as we go. Keep in mind that as you tense each muscle group, you should use your energy to hold the muscle tight, but you do not need to strain yourself. If there are any muscle groups that are particularly sore or if you are unable for any reason to tense a particular muscle group, just continue with your deep breathing and general relaxation through that muscle group. Try to focus on recognizing the difference between how your muscles feel when they are tense and how they feel when they are relaxed.

Now tighten the muscles in your feet by pointing your toes away from you. Hold the tension for a moment in the arch of your foot, the top of your foot, and your calf. Hold that position as you count in your mind along with me: one, two, three, four, five, six, seven, eight, nine, ten. Now squeeze so your muscles are just a little bit tighter . . . and then release. Enjoy the sensations of relaxation in your feet and lower legs. Take a deep breath in through your nose and then slowly breathe out, being sure to allow any tension in your feet or legs to just drain away. Just drain away. (Repeat this tense and release cycle one time.) Rest now and enjoy the sensation of having your feet and lower legs release and relax. Think quietly to yourself as you breathe, "I am relaxed and comfortable." Great job.

Next we're going to focus on your lower legs. Tighten your calf muscles by flexing your toes up so they are pointing at your head. Hold the tension in your calves and count with me: one, two, three, four, five, six, seven, eight, nine, ten. Now squeeze so your muscles are just a little bit tighter. Hold it . . . and then release. Focus on the sensations of relaxation in your lower legs, your ankles, and your feet. Take a deep breath in through your nose and then slowly breathe out, being sure to allow any tension in your lower legs to just drain away. Just drain away. (Repeat this tense and release cycle one time.) Rest now and enjoy the sensation of having your lower legs release and relax. Think quietly to yourself as you breathe, "I am relaxed and comfortable." Excellent.

Now we're going to focus on your upper legs. Squeeze the muscles in your thighs down to your knees. To do this, you will also need to tighten the muscles in your hips, the top of your thighs, and the bottom of your thighs. Hold the tension in your legs and count with me: one, two, three, four, five, six, seven, eight, nine, ten. Now squeeze so your muscles are just a little bit tighter . . . and then release. Enjoy the sensations of relaxation in your upper legs from your hips all the way down to your knees. Take a deep breath in and then slowly breathe out, being sure to allow any remaining tension in your legs to just drain away. (Repeat this tense and release cycle one time.) Rest now and enjoy the sensation of having your thighs and hips release and relax. Think quietly to yourself as you breathe, "I am relaxed and comfortable." Notice how still and relaxed your legs have become.

Now hold both of your arms out straight in front of you, lock your elbows, and clench your fists. Hold the tension in your arms and fists as tightly as you possibly can. Hold it for one, two, three, four, five, six, seven, eight, nine, ten. Now squeeze so your muscles are just a little bit tighter. Good. And then release. Allow your arms to fall back to your side with your palms facing up and allow the fingers in your hands to relax and uncurl. Enjoy the sensations of relaxation in your arms, hands, and fingers. Take a deep breath in and then slowly breathe out, being sure to allow any muscle tension in your arms or hands to just drain away. (Repeat this tense and release cycle one time.) Excellent. Notice now how limp and relaxed your arms and hands feel. Perhaps they also feel light or tingly, or warm or heavy. Take a deep breath and enjoy this pleasant sensation, whatever it may be for you.

Now tighten your biceps, the muscles between your shoulders and your elbows, by bringing your forearms up toward your shoulders as if you were making a muscle with both arms. Squeeze your fists and hold the tension in your biceps while you count with me: one, two, three, four, five, six, seven, eight, nine, ten. Now squeeze so your muscles are just a little bit tighter . . . and then release. Again, allow your arms to fall back to your side with your palms facing up and let the fingers in your hands relax and uncurl. Enjoy the sensations of relaxation in your biceps and shoulders. Take a deep breath in and then slowly breathe out, being sure to allow any muscle tension in your biceps or shoulders to just drain away. (Repeat this tense and release cycle one time.) Rest now and enjoy the sensation of having your bicep muscles release and relax. Great job.

Now we're going to focus on the muscles in your back. Tilt your head back, so that you have a gentle stretch on the front of your neck, arch your back, stick out your belly, and try to bring your shoulder blades together behind you as you maintain this stretch. Count in your mind one, two, three, four, five, six, seven, eight, nine, ten. Now squeeze just a little bit tighter. Hold it . . . and then release. Enjoy the sensations of relaxation in your back and shoulders. Take a deep breath in and then slowly breathe out, being sure to allow any remaining tension in your back and shoulders to just drain away. (Repeat this tense and release cycle one time.) Rest now and enjoy the sensation of comfort in your back and shoulders. Think quietly to yourself as you breathe and rest, "I am relaxed and comfortable."

Now tighten your neck and shoulders by shrugging your shoulders all the way up to your ears. Hold the tension in your shoulders and neck, and count with me: one, two, three, four, five, six, seven, eight, nine, ten. Now squeeze so your muscles are just a little bit tighter. And then release. Allow your shoulders to fall back to their neutral position and relax your neck, upper back, and shoulders. Enjoy the sensations of relaxation in your neck and shoulders. Take a deep breath in and then slowly breathe out, being sure to allow any muscle tension in your neck, back, and shoulders to just drain away. (Repeat this tense and release cycle one time.) Rest now and enjoy the sensation of having your neck, back, and shoulders release and relax. Great job.

Next we're going to tighten the muscles in your face by squeezing your eyelids tightly shut and clenching your jaw. Hold the tension all around your eyes, forehead, cheeks, and jaw and count with me: one, two, three, four, five, six, seven, eight, nine, ten. Now squeeze so your muscles are just a little bit tighter . . . and then release. Enjoy the sensations of relaxation in your eyes, all around your forehead, across the top of your head, and through your cheeks and jaw. Take a deep breath and then slowly breathe out, being sure to allow any tension in your face to just drain away. (Repeat this tense and release cycle one time.) Rest now and enjoy the sensation of having your face, eyes, and jaw release and relax. Think quietly to yourself, "I am relaxed and comfortable." Perfect.

Next we're going to focus on releasing the muscles in your jaw. Open your mouth so wide that it feels you cannot open the hinges of your jaw any wider. Hold your mouth open as wide as you can and count with me: one, two, three, four, five, six, seven, eight, nine, ten. Now open just a little bit bigger . . . and then release. Notice the sensations of relaxation in your jaw, cheeks, and neck. Take a deep breath in and then slowly breathe out, being sure to allow any remaining tension in your jaw, cheeks, or neck to just drain away. (Repeat this tense and release cycle one time.) Rest now and enjoy the sensation of having your jaw and neck release and relax. Think quietly to yourself as you breathe, "I am relaxed and comfortable." Notice how still your body has become. You are doing wonderfully.

Now I invite you to close your eyes if they are not already closed. Imagine for a moment that you are floating on a raft in a warm ocean. Feel the waves pass beneath you as you are gently rocked from your head down to your toes. You are floating up and over a gentle wave and then back down, rocking from your head down to your toes. With each gentle wave you feel more and more relaxed. Up and over the waves, you rock in the warm ocean. Feel the water and the waves wash over you. Each wave drains more and more tension from your body.

Now that you've completely soothed your body, just enjoy this feeling for the next minute. At the end of one minute you will hear my voice again (wait one minute). Wonderful job.

Stay Awake Ending

I will now slowly count backwards from five to one. When I reach one you can choose to open your eyes feeling rested, alert, relaxed, and very comfortable. Five . . . four . . . three . . . two . . . one.

Go to Sleep Ending

I will now slowly count backwards from five to one. When I reach one you may gently drift off into a deep and comfortable sleep. Five . . . four . . . three . . . two . . . one.

SCRIPT FOR PASSIVE PROGRESSIVE MUSCLE RELAXATION

Take a few slow, deep breaths to get started. Breathe in through your nose and out through your mouth. Just pace yourself in a way that feels comfortable, smooth, and easy. Breathe in through your nose, pulling the air down into your belly, pause for just a moment, then breathe your air out through your mouth. With each breath in, you are becoming more and more relaxed. With each breath out, you are feeling more and more calm and comfortable. Slow and steady, releasing any tension. Relax now and give your body time to heal. Relax and know that this is just what you are supposed to do.

Now close your eyes so your mind can do its best work. Imagine a soft, soothing color. Any color you wish. Pour this color into an empty paint can. Next imagine that you have a soft paintbrush. Dip this paintbrush into your soothing color and gently brush it on your right foot. As it touches your foot, feel the soothing quality of the paint. Imagine that it releases any muscle tension you may feel in your foot and helps it to feel very comfortable. Next, gently stroke the paintbrush up your right leg. It may take a couple of strokes to cover your leg completely. Take your time. As you cover your leg with this soft, soothing color, feel the muscles relax and the pleasant feelings increase. Notice that your leg may feel warmer, heavier, and more relaxed. Next brush your left foot with this soothing, healing color. Feel the paintbrush gently stroke the bottom of your foot and pass over the top of your foot. Allow the paintbrush to continue up your shin and thigh, covering all of your left leg with this soft, soothing color. Notice now how relaxed your legs feel. Notice how this color may have changed the sensation in your legs.

Now pass this paintbrush dipped in your soothing color over the palm of your right hand and up over each one of your fingertips. Allow the brush to move up to your wrist, forearm, and to the top of your arm. Now dip and swish the brush in your soothing color and apply it to your right shoulder. As you do, feel your shoulder relax and notice how calm and still your right arm and shoulder now feel.

Now the paintbrush slowly moves over to your left hand. Feel the soft bristles gently stroke the palm of your left hand and then pass over each of your fingertips. Watch as the soothing color covers your left wrist, forearm, and the top of your arm, and notice now that all of your limbs feel warm, heavy, and relaxed. Cover the paintbrush in your soothing color and cover your left shoulder with this color so that it too becomes heavy and relaxed.

Now pass this paintbrush up the back of your neck, the back of your head and top of your head. Feel your scalp gently tingle and relax. Pass the soft brush over your forehead, nose, eyes, cheeks, and chin. Notice how all the tension just drains from your face. Take a deep breath in and enjoy this feeling of relaxation.

Next pass the paintbrush down your chest and across your stomach. Feel your breathing deepen and your muscles in your chest and belly relax. Feel the tension just drain away.

Now take a moment to scan your body. If there is any place that is not completely relaxed and comfortable, gently pass the paintbrush dipped in your soothing color back and forth over that particular area. Back and forth, back and forth, releasing discomfort and tension. You are feeling more and more relaxed. You have as much of your soothing color as you need to make your body feel comfortable. Take your time. Focus on your breath and on releasing any leftover stress or tension in your body. As the brush passes back and forth, back and forth, you feel more and more relaxed.

Stay Awake Ending

Now that you've completely soothed your body, you can return to feeling awake and focused and you can take these relaxing feelings with you. I will slowly count backward from five to one. When I reach one, you can open your eyes feeling rested, alert, relaxed, and very comfortable. Five . . . four . . . three . . . two . . . one.

Go to Sleep Ending

I'm going to count down from ten slowly and when I reach one, you can peacefully drift off into a deep and comfortable sleep.
10 . . . 9 . . . 8 . . . Feeling calm and relaxed
7 . . . 6 . . . 5 . . . Easing slowly into sleep
4 . . . 3 . . . 2 . . . More and more relaxed
1 . . . Resting gently as you drift quietly to sleep.

◆

How to Help

1. EXPLAIN THE EXERCISE TO YOUR CHILD

Tell your child that the exercise you want to try will help to relieve muscle tension throughout the body. Explain that tensing a muscle signals to the brain that an area of the body is calling for oxygen-rich blood and that tensing and then releasing a muscle can help sore, tired, or achy muscles to heal. Make it clear that these exercises can help kids to feel more deeply relaxed from head to toe.

2. PREPARE YOUR CHILD

Have your child stretch out on a bed, couch, or on the floor. If you are doing an active muscle relaxation where you will instruct your child to tense each muscle group, be sure your child has removed his or her shoes and is not wearing overly tight or restrictive clothing.

3. MAKE PRACTICING A PRIORITY

Similar to guided imagery, this is a skill that requires practice. Set aside ten to fifteen minutes of time *each day* to practice, and be sure to put away cell phones and other distractions. Let other family members know that you can't be disturbed until you have completed the practice. Don't give up too easily. Even though many kids could do this exercise on their own, parent support and guidance can go a long way toward reinforcing the benefit and encouraging good practice habits, especially in the beginning. Keep in mind that daily practices can lead to a generally more relaxed body (and mind), and so may help to prevent muscle tightness and pain.

4. COMBINE WITH GUIDED IMAGERY OR OTHER RELAXATION STRATEGIES

Children or adolescents who have trouble settling in for guided-imagery work often benefit from starting with a progressive muscle relaxation. The concrete experience of the muscle relaxation exercise is very appealing to kids, and the contrast between tense and relaxed muscles is almost always immediately noticeable. Once they are relaxed in this way, many children can more effectively engage in guided-imagery exercises. For some great apps designed to help with progressive muscle relaxation and other relaxation strategies, see Appendix 3.

13

One Mindful Moment at a Time

Mindfulness is the act of purposefully paying very close attention to one's present experience. When practicing mindfulness, a person thinks about what is going on *now*. When you think only about the present moment, you can't also be thinking about tomorrow, or next week, or five years from now, or the million other things that race (or meander) through your mind. For example, think for a moment only about the place where you are sitting. What do you notice about the surface? What do you notice about the walls or ceiling around you? What sensation do you have in your fingertips at the moment? What noises or sounds do you hear? By focusing your attention on the experiences you are having right now, you are choosing to not pay attention to unpleasant thoughts or experiences such as discomfort, fear, worry, stress, or sadness. We know that focusing on pain or discomfort can lead to more pain and discomfort. Fortunately, the opposite is also true. Choosing to focus one's mind on other "in-the-moment" sensations can reduce physical discomfort and emotional distress.

In addition to staying focused in the present moment, an important component of mindfulness includes a willingness to remain open-minded. The goal is to approach present experiences, whatever they may be, with an accepting attitude and a natural curiosity. This positive framework enhances the experience of mindfulness and ensures that all present-minded experiences can be accepted openly.

Mindfulness is a meditative practice that originated in Buddhism, but it has gained significant popularity in the Western world due to its research-proven ability to induce feelings of calm, increase feelings of self-efficacy, and help people of all ages manage stress and negative experiences. Many pain-management practitioners have welcomed mindfulness techniques because they know that they can greatly reduce pain-related distress, making it possible for people to be more active and engaged in their lives.

Here's an example of how mindfulness can work. I recently met with John, a sixteen-year-old boy with multiple pain problems. Upon entering my office he reported that he had a horrible headache with pounding, exploding pressure in his ears and so much tightness across his forehead that he thought his head was going to crack open. His heart was also racing and he was breathing with short, shallow breaths. He thought his symptoms meant that his blood pressure was too high, and he was very worried that he was going to have a heart attack or stroke right then and there. Because I knew John well, and knew that he was not at risk for a heart attack or stroke, I was able to use mindfulness strategies to help diffuse the situation.

I started by asking John to take three deep breaths and then to report the sensations he was experiencing without assigning any judgment to them. This is mindfulness work. He had to tell me what he was experiencing in the moment, but he had to leave out all of the negative or scary words and worries and simply describe the sensations. With this in mind, he reported, "I feel a lot of pressure in my ears. It feels like I'm underwater. I also have tightness across my forehead and my chest feels tight." We then discussed that pressure in the ears is not inherently bad; it's just a sensation. We further discussed that if he was swimming in a pool, the pressure or underwater sensation would probably seem normal and not at all scary or uncomfortable. Immediately, he began to relax. We talked about how if he were wearing a scuba mask strapped across his forehead, the sensation of tightness would also not seem so bad. By acknowledging the sensation without passing judgment about the experience, he could see that while he was uncomfortable, his symptoms were not intolerable.

I then proceeded to use a guided-imagery technique (see Chapter 11) to make his brain feel as if he was actually swimming in a clear blue lagoon on a hot summer day. The "as if" feeling we created of water against his ears normalized the sensation of pressure on his ears and this further reduced his anxiety and helped him to recognize that his symptoms were not inherently scary. We also used a scuba mask visualization in the guided imagery to normalize the sensation of tightness across his forehead. He was then able to visualize loosening the scuba mask to relieve the tension, which further helped him to relax and decrease the symptoms. We visualized that the chest tightness was due to his holding his breath underwater and I described how he could surface in the lagoon, breathing out deeply and then inhaling fresh clean air into his relaxed chest. Once he recognized that he could experience sensations (such as pressure in his ears, or tightness on his forehead and chest) without worry, fear, or negativity (his fear of an exploding head, too-high blood pressure, or imminent stroke), his stress was greatly reduced. By using a mindfulness approach to the present sensation in his body (along with a combination of deep breathing and guided imagery), he could relax enough within just ten minutes to greatly alleviate his uncomfortable headache.

Mindfulness work can include a focus on cognitive experiences such as present thoughts and emotions, as well as sensory experiences like sights, sounds, touch, scent, or taste. The goal is to bring full awareness to our immediate experience, and to do so without determining whether the experience is good or bad. By electing to actively focus on a present thought or experience, a person is in essence blocking the brain's ability to focus on anything else.

Mindfulness with kids can actually be very fun and engaging. One of my favorite ways to teach mindfulness with children and adolescents is to focus on non-pain-related sensory experiences, which are more concrete than internal feelings and experiences and so a bit easier to be mindful about. Older adolescents, however, can certainly focus on more internal processes, especially once they have been introduced to the practice.

How to Practice Mindfulness

The easiest way to teach mindfulness to kids is through concrete experiments. For example, mindfulness-based touching can be taught by either blindfolding your child or having your child close his eyes and placing an object in his hand. Ask your child to touch the object and try to describe it without naming the object and without using judgments. For example, if touching a piece of velvet, try not to describe it by saying, "This feels good; it's velvet." Instead, say, "This is a small piece of fabric that feels smooth when I rub it in one direction and rough when I rub in the other direction." Talk with your child about how describing things experienced through touch is different from naming or judging them. The process of actively observing and describing is much more engaging and distracting. Encourage your child to maintain a curious approach to the experiment. You can also try mindfulness-based visual experiments by playing the game "I never noticed." Use simple objects around the home, interesting details about people's faces, a patch of grass outside, and so on. Have your child try to expand his or her awareness so that she can name ten things she hadn't noticed before being mindful. You can do the same thing with hearing. Work with your child to see what you can hear when you mindfully allocate all of your attention to sound.

Of all the mindfulness-based sensory experiences, my favorite mindfulness practice with kids is mindful tasting or eating. Being mindful with food is very interesting and fun for children, especially when it involves a treat. The goal is to have a child examine and savor the food and experience a favorite food in a whole new way.

When I teach my pain-management workshop to adolescents, I lead a mindfulness-based practice of eating a chocolate kiss. The kids love the experiment. Somewhat predictably, parents started to complain that they couldn't truly understand the experiment unless they tried it themselves. I couldn't argue with that logic. So now the parents get to practice mindfully eating a chocolate kiss as well. When I ask parents to share about their experience, the most common remark is, "That was the best chocolate kiss I ever ate." When all of your attention is allocated to an eating experience, you appreciate the food more intensely. By using mindfulness we were able to greatly elevate the experience of eating the often-underappreciated chocolate kiss from a "ho-hum" experience to a "best chocolate kiss ever" experience.

Below is an example script for a chocolate mindfulness practice for you and your child to do together. If you or your child doesn't eat chocolate, you can try this experiment with gummy bears, skittles, dried fruit, ice, popcorn, peanut butter, or anything else both of you love to eat. It can enhance the experience if you practice this while listening to soft, relaxing music or using white noise to block out noise in the background.

SCRIPT FOR EATING MINDFULLY

Touch the piece of chocolate.

Pay attention to the shape and feel of the chocolate.

Notice smooth and rough features.

Notice when the chocolate warms in your hand and some of the outside edges start to soften and melt.

Deeply inhale to smell the chocolate and notice how you now start to crave the experience of tasting the chocolate in your mouth.

Gently place one bite of chocolate on your tongue and close your mouth. Do not let the chocolate touch the roof of your mouth; just experience it on your tongue.

Notice how your mouth begins to salivate in anticipation of eating the chocolate.

Be aware of the flavor experience building in your mouth.

Notice the sweetness when you next swallow.

Now slowly press the chocolate to the roof of your mouth.

Notice the change in the intensity of the flavor.

Swirl the now-melting chocolate around in your mouth and enjoy the flavors and sensations.

Work toward making your experience with this piece of chocolate last as long as possible.

Savor. Enjoy. Savor. Enjoy.

When the chocolate has completely dissolved, notice the taste left in your mouth. Pay attention to your emotional experience. How is your mood after savoring this delicious piece of chocolate?

When the experience of the first bite of chocolate has finally passed, try this experience with the second bite of chocolate.

See what you can notice that is different about the chocolate the second time around.

Challenge your mind and body to make this experience even longer and more intense than the first experience. Notice the calm and comfort you feel after focusing your mind and fully enjoying this experience.

WALKING MINDFULLY

Beyond the sensory exploration of mindfulness, I've found that children really enjoy walking-based mindfulness practices. Walking exercises, sometimes called walking meditations, take a lot of "in-the-moment" energy, and for that reason are excellent at keeping kids focused on the present moment. For example, ask your child to walk exactly twenty paces in a straight line. Talk about how hard that was or how much attention that took. Next make a straight line on the floor with a piece of tape and have your child try to walk twenty paces without stepping off the taped line. Remind your child to keep an open and accepting frame of mind, so that when he falls off the line he can remain calm, take a deep breath to help gather his concentration, and continue. Once your child has mastered walking on the taped straight line, have him try to walk the line with his eyes closed. Or you can give your child a full-to-the-brim cup of water and have her try to walk the line without spilling the water. Talk to your child about this experiment. How much attention did each part take? What else was going through her mind? When your child was more focused on the present moment task, did she notice fewer extraneous thoughts?

Another walking mindfulness experiment that I call "sticky feet" emphasizes the importance of moving forward, even in a challenging situation. The goal is to have your child imagine that he or she has very sticky soles on his or her feet. This experience is about focusing on staying grounded and making small steps in the right direction.

Follow these steps and try this exercise along with your child.

1. Imagine that your feet are sticky on the bottom, as if covered in glue. The only way to keep from getting stuck completely is to continue slowly moving forward.
2. Place one foot down on the ground, heel to toe. Feel your foot make contact with the ground and focus on the sensation of slowly lifting each foot and moving steadily forward.
3. Go as slowly as possible at first. Remember to breathe deeply as you move. With each breath, reward your body for making progress.
4. With each small step, pay attention to the way in which your feet carry your body. Notice the shift in weight from the heel, to the mid-foot, to the toes. Roll off the toes slowly into the next step.
5. Feel grounded in the present moment. Notice how your feet stay firmly attached to the ground and continue to support you as you move forward.
6. If you become aware of other thoughts or sensations, return your attention to the strength in your feet, and notice the success you are making as you move forward slowly and steadily, always breathing, always moving.
7. Notice that no matter what experiences you have, your sticky feet will keep you grounded, keep you solid and keep you mindfully moving forward.

THINKING MINDFULLY

Another exercise that fits well within the practice of mindfulness is a cognitive strategy known as floating. The idea behind floating is to remain in the moment and to rise, or float, above ongoing stressors, difficulties, or discomforts. The goal is to acknowledge the difficulty, but not allow oneself to be bothered by whatever it might be. Floating is about learning how to accept challenging situations and float right over them. Whether a difficulty is pain-related or due to other challenges such as peer or school stress, sometimes children just need a way to get over and past the issue. Teaching your child how to float over these difficulties, instead of letting each difficulty stand in the way, can help empower her to manage stressful situations. The next script, about an ice cream float, is designed to be read by a parent to a child, though you can paraphrase or embellish it as you wish. Even better, make an ice cream float with your child and then, while enjoying it together, explain this mindfulness approach.

The Ice Cream Float

Let's learn to make your mind float like a scoop of ice cream atop a fizzy soda. Think about what an ice cream float looks like. There is fizzy soda on the bottom and a scoop of cool ice cream bobbing on top. Notice how the ice cream just floats on top of the soda. All the fizz from the soda bubbles up and provides the lift so that the ice cream can enjoy bouncing on top, not at all bothered by what's underneath.

You can be like this ice cream. Imagine that your next stressful or uncomfortable situation is like the fizzy soda and you are like the scoop of ice cream. You are just bouncing along the top of the experience and not at all concerned with the details or depths of the situation.

Imagine that you are well supported in your present moment and even though you know there is a lot going on beneath you (where all that fizzy soda is), you don't have to be bothered by it at all. Isn't it nice to know that you can stay cool in the present moment (just like the ice cream) and float across the top of whatever experience you choose? And here's an interesting part: if you could observe an ice cream float that didn't get eaten right away, you'd notice that the ice cream slowly starts to melt or dissolve into the fizzy soda. You would also observe that the soda becomes less fizzy over time. It's just like dealing with a challenge in life: often after floating for a bit over an uncomfortable or difficult situation, you may find that you don't feel as bothered by the situation anymore.

ACTING MINDFULLY

Acting mindfully is about bringing acts of gratitude and compassion into the present moment. When a child or family is consumed with pain, stress, or other challenges, it is very easy to lose sight of the many things for which one is grateful. Acting mindfully is about making choices that have positive implications for other individuals as well as within the greater communities of family, school, neighborhoods, and cities. While it's easy to delay acting mindfully when one is consumed by worry, stress, or physical challenges, focusing on the actions that make a positive difference in the lives of others can be a significant part of the healing and coping process.

Encourage your child to engage in an experience that will expand his or her awareness beyond him- or herself. Take your child to volunteer at an animal shelter or food bank, assign your child to make dinner for the family one night, or have your child ask the neighbors if they need help in the yard or with another task and have your child complete this without pay. Acting mindfully in this way not only is a great way to teach kindness and compassion, but also provides your child with feelings of accomplishment, pride, and self-efficacy—which can be hard to come by when children are struggling to cope with chronic pain.

Staying in the Moment

Mindfulness doesn't have to be complicated. In fact, the simpler the strategy, the more consistent it is with a mindfulness framework. You might try some of the following fun ideas the next time you're looking for ways to encourage your child's own mindfulness practice.

WRITING YOUR NAME IN THE PALM OF YOUR HAND

When your child is stressed or uncomfortable, teach your child to focus on the pleasant sensation of drawing lightly on the palm of his or her own hand. Your child can write the letters of their first, middle, and last name or draw a favorite shape. As an added challenge, have your child close his or her eyes and you can draw something in your child's palm. Have your child try to guess what you drew.

FINGER-TAPPING MANTRA

Work with your child to come up with a five-word mantra that inspires or motivates your child. Examples include "I am strong and healthy," "I can rise above this," "Pain does not control me" "I'm calm and at peace," "My mind is all mine," "Thinking calm thoughts right now," or "I know I am loved." Once your child decides on a five-word mantra, assign one word to each finger on your child's left or right hand. Have your child practice saying each word to herself as she taps each finger in succession on her thigh or on a table. This exercise can help to soothe your child in any circumstance. Parents can also tap this out on their child as a special, inconspicuous way of communicating care and concern during a particularly stressful time. Combine this exercise with deep breathing for an added benefit. Simply breathe in the first word, breath out the second word, breathe in the third word, and so on. This slows the tapping down considerably and encourages a mindful focus on breathing.

◆

How to Help

1. EXPLAIN MINDFULNESS TO YOUR CHILD

Tell your child that the practice of mindfulness involves thinking and feeling about what is happening right now. Emphasize that an important part of mindfulness is keeping an open, curious mind and not talking about feelings or sensations as being good or bad. The focus is on being aware of the present moment.

2. PRACTICE EVERYWHERE

Mindfulness is a truly always-accessible comfort strategy. In the beginning you will have to prompt your child to stay in the present moment. But soon you and your child will likely find that it is very enjoyable to remain open, curious, and present-minded in your day-to-day activities. Wake up, look out the window, and notice the shifting shape of clouds in the sky; listen mindfully to the crunch of your morning cereal; learn how many steps it takes to get from the kitchen to the car; and so on. Teach your child that mindfulness can steer one's awareness away from stress or pain so that the focus can be on experiences that evoke more positive thoughts and feelings.

3. STAY POSITIVE

Cultivating mindfulness can take time. At first a mindfulness practice may last only two minutes. That's completely fine. As your child builds more skill for staying focused in the present, he will be able to expand the length of his practice. When your child slips into comments about future worries, current negative experiences of pain, or concerns from the past, simply acknowledge the comment, saying something like, "I understand that you are hurting right now. Let's stay focused in the present for one more minute by trying. . . ." Be positive in your approach so there is never a feeling of failure. We want to protect children's positive feelings about mindfulness so that they will be motivated to use it whenever they need it in their struggles to overcome chronic pain.

4. POINT OUT THE DIFFERENCE BETWEEN MINDFULNESS AND AVOIDANCE

I once had an adolescent really latch on to the idea of mindfulness. She came to our therapy session one day and let me know that she wasn't able to follow through with the plan to get back to school because thinking about that future event made her anxious. She instead continued to not think about it by staying home and practicing mindfulness. Unfortunately, she confused mindfulness with not carrying out a plan intended to help in her overall recovery. To be clear, avoidance is not doing things that cause stress, anxiety, or discomfort. Mindfulness, by contrast, is acknowledging that there is stress, anxiety, or discomfort and using a present-minded focus to reduce distress so that you can still do what you need to do. My patient was commended for her keen interest in mindfulness, and then instructed how to use her mindfulness skills to reduce the unpleasant feelings of stress and anxiety when she got on the bus for school the next day.

14
Biofeedback

Pain and stress both trigger the sympathetic nervous system, which in response will automatically prepare the body for "fight or flight." A person feeling pain or stress will thus commonly experience physiological changes such as an increased heart rate, shallow breathing, elevated blood pressure, slowed digestion, decreased blood flow to the extremities, and increased muscle tension—all in preparation for running away or mounting a defense. Relaxation exercises like diaphragmatic breathing, guided imagery, progressive muscle relaxation, and mindfulness are explicitly designed to activate the parasympathetic nervous system response, otherwise known as the relaxation response. The parasympathetic system overrides the sympathetic activity, and so will reduce blood pressure, slow the heart rate, restore digestive function, increase blood flow to the extremities, and relax the muscles—in other words, it will restore the body to a healthier state. But how do you or your child really know if the parasympathetic systems are fully engaged and helping? In other words, how do you know if the relaxation exercises are working?

One way to know for sure if your child is triggering the relaxation response is to talk to your child about how he or she feels. If your child feels relaxed, soothed, less stressed, more focused, or more comfortable after engaging in any relaxation exercise, then you know that it's working. You can also observe your child's response. If your child is focused and engaged and actively participates with you in these activities, then you should be assured that he or she will benefit from them. But if either you or your child is uncertain, or if you have a difficult time engaging your child in relaxation work, then it may be worthwhile to consider a biofeedback approach.

What Is Biofeedback?

The word biofeedback simply denotes getting information ("feedback") from the body ("bio"). The term first became popular in the late 1960s. At that time biofeedback was used to describe laboratory procedures that trained research subjects to alter their own brain activity, blood pressure, muscle tension, heart rate, and other bodily functions that are not normally controlled voluntarily. Over the last fifty years, due in part to a robust research literature supporting the efficacy of this technique, biofeedback has moved out of the laboratory and into mainstream culture. Currently the term is used to describe a mind-body training technique in which people are taught to improve their health and physical performance by using signals from their own bodies. Biofeedback, or biofeedback-assisted relaxation therapy (BART), essentially helps people learn how to gain control over the automatic nervous system by showing them the physiological differences between the activated sympathetic nervous system and the relaxed parasympathetic response.

Biofeedback involves equipment that takes real-time assessments of internal body functions such as heart rate, breath rate, muscle contraction, or temperature and makes them outwardly observable. A simple medical device such as a thermometer is essentially a biofeedback tool, because it provides information that allows a person to make a health-related decision. For example if a thermometer reveals that a person's body temperature is high, she may decide to hydrate, rest, or take medication until symptoms resolve. The goal with biofeedback is simply to obtain data from the body and respond in a way that will promote relief.

Biofeedback devices used in pain management and stress reduction commonly measure heart rate, breath rate, skin conductance (the amount of moisture produced by the fingertips), external temperature, and muscle tension. Years ago the equipment used in the clinical practice of biofeedback was very expensive, and often quite cumbersome and complicated. But as the practice of biofeedback has grown and technologies have improved, the equipment used by providers has become more streamlined and user-friendly. Most often, biofeedback procedures involve attaching sensors to the fingertips or skin to assess heart rate, external temperature, and skin conductance; attaching soft, expandable tubing around the chest and diaphragm to assess breath rate; or applying sticky pads to muscles to assess muscle tension. All sensors are connected to wires that feed into a computer or device and then display, via visual and/or auditory cues, information in real-time about an activity. Biofeedback is not at all uncomfortable, and in fact most kids really enjoy the experience.

Biofeedback has been validated as a successful treatment tool for a wide variety of health-related difficulties. There is good empirical support for the use of biofeedback to treat headache (tension and migraine), temporomandibular disorders (TMJ), Raynaud's disease (poor circulation), high blood pressure, chronic pain, anxiety disorders, postural orthostatic tachycardia syndrome (POTS), fibromyalgia, and stroke recovery or Bell's palsy (muscle re-education). Additionally, when you consider that biofeedback is simply a tool to enhance learning about the relaxation response, it's easy to understand how this could be a useful strategy for anyone who wants to learn relaxation.

I frequently tell my patients that it's not necessary to use biofeedback for pain management, but it can be a very helpful part of a therapeutic plan. Biofeedback makes relaxation very concrete and understandable and so can be especially useful for children who are resistant to the idea of relaxation as a way to manage pain. With biofeedback equipment, real-time changes are visualized on a display. So when I'm working with a child doing biofeedback I can say, "I know you are breathing deeply, but I can see on my computer that you are not relaxing your shoulders. Let's try actively releasing tension there and see how that helps you to relax more deeply." When that child responds by releasing her shoulder tension, she can immediately see the change on the display. Seeing the change on the screen and associating that change with the positive feelings of relaxation helps children gain confidence in their ability to control their own bodies. When a child sees that she can control her own heart rate, breathing, muscle tension, temperature, and other physiological processes, she may become more motivated to integrate relaxation work into her day-to-day management of pain and pain-related stress.

Another benefit of biofeedback is that it's engaging and fun for kids. When trying to improve a child's self-efficacy in managing pain, we sometimes need all the bells and whistles we can get. If kids like the interactive games or are interested in the science behind biofeedback, it further enhances their engagement, motivation, and willingness to practice relaxation techniques.

Basic biofeedback tools can be used with children as young as age six. Younger children may simply have trouble understanding the meaning of the biofeedback signal and so may find making adjustments too challenging. There are truly no identifiable risks to trying biofeedback. Some children do not like biofeedback because they may feel in some way that their relaxation efforts are being judged or tested. This feeling of being evaluated leads to increased anxiety, which certainly interferes with the intended benefits.

Biofeedback can be done by a variety of health providers including psychologists, physical therapists, and nurses. The techniques and equipment may vary somewhat depending on the professional who is leading the practice, but the foundation of the practice, which includes both obtaining a biofeedback signal and providing a skilled in-the-moment interpretation of the signal for the patient, is generally the same no matter who leads the session.

When working with a health care professional, biofeedback is typically integrated into a more comprehensive framework. For example, I use biofeedback as a way to show children how they can be effective when engaging in behaviorally based relaxation exercises such as guided imagery and progressive muscle relaxation. I can also use biofeedback to demonstrate the powerful influence that our thoughts have on our physiology. For example, while a child is connected to a biofeedback device that assesses heart rate and skin conductance, I frequently invite him or her to tell me about an embarrassing moment. Telling this story causes an immediate increase in heart rate and skin conductance. I can then use this data as a launch pad for a discussion about how our thoughts affect our nervous system, even when we are not noticing that this is happening. To reverse this autonomic nervous system arousal, I then help the child practice diaphragmatic breathing or mindfulness and the two of us watch in real time as the parasympathetic nervous system kicks in, triggering the relaxation response and restoring the heart rate and skin conductance to baseline (or better).

Biofeedback Basics

Because an increasing number of providers are integrating biofeedback tools into clinical practice for pain management and because some biofeedback tools are readily available for home use, it's useful for parents to understand a few key elements of biofeedback. First and foremost, with all biofeedback, the change in the biofeedback signal is the most important element, not the absolute value of the signal. For example, muscle tension is measured in microvolts. When I'm working with a child to teach muscle relaxation, I don't focus much on the baseline microvolt measurement; instead I care about how much they are able to lower it. Specifically, I'm looking for changes in physiology that indicate the muscles are changing from a state of tension to one of relaxation.

Another important element in biofeedback is the suggestion for *how* to change the signal. I might suggest to a child to try five diaphragmatic breaths and we would watch the display to see if that changed the signal. If not, then we might try to pair diaphragmatic breathing with a

171

ten-minute guided-imagery exercise to see if that improved the signal. If that approach was successful, I would suggest that the child practice diaphragmatic breathing in combination with guided imagery at home because that is what produced the best results during our practice.

The last important element to practicing biofeedback is reinforcement. Most biofeedback tools have built-in reinforcements. For example, one biofeedback game I use in treatment has an image on-screen of a far-off mountain with the mountain peak hidden in the clouds. Each successful diaphragmatic breath the child completes is rewarded on-screen with the magical appearance of a single stair. Each successive stair is linked to the previous one to build a golden bridge that climbs into the sky toward the mountain. As the bridge gets closer to the mountain, the clouds part, revealing a golden temple. Successful completion of the bridge is followed by a cascade of music and a video in which the viewer seems to soar over the bridge into the temple. The built-in reinforcement is critical for successful biofeedback; it lets the user know when he or she needs to make adjustments. For example, when steps do not magically appear, it signals that the user may need to try breathing more deeply, thinking more positive thoughts, or finding other ways to reduce tension. When the user has successfully attained steps, it means that his or her relaxation efforts have been effective.

Beyond the built-in reinforcement of biofeedback systems, positive reinforcement from parents and health professionals is also very important. One biofeedback system I use has a color-coded reinforcement graph. When a child is tense, the graph is yellow. As the child becomes more relaxed, the color changes from yellow to green to blue. Bright blue indicates that the child has attained a physiological state of relaxation. If I were working with a child suffering from chronic tension headaches, I might interpret and reinforce this signal by saying something like:

Maintaining a slow and steady breath makes your body more relaxed. Notice that it only took you a few moments to become relaxed enough to get into the "blue range" today. That's great! It took much longer when you first started. When your body is in the "blue range" it is in a state of relaxation. Getting to the "blue range" means you are actively reducing the tension in your body. Remember that tension is what contributes to your headaches. If you relax your body like this throughout the day, you may discover you have fewer headaches. So, as you are relaxing right now, pay attention to how your body feels so you can re-create this "blue range" feeling at home.

There are many biofeedback systems currently available. Parents should keep in mind that there is wide variation in terms of biofeedback programs' reliability and overall quality. When the programs are sensitive to changes in biorhythms they can be very helpful, but if they are unreliable or not sensitive enough to small changes, the process can be frustrating, especially for children. Even so, many high-quality, inexpensive biofeedback tools are available for in-home use. For example, for fewer than five dollars you can purchase a biofeedback card, similar in size and shape to a credit card, that includes a temperature-sensitive piece of plastic, not unlike the material found in mood rings, that changes color in different temperatures. Your child can hold this simple card in his or her hand while practicing relaxation techniques and try to turn the card from black to blue to green, indicating various degrees of relaxation. Other inexpensive biofeedback tools include digital peripheral thermometers and even some engaging, fun applications for smartphones.

◆

How to Help

1. TALK WITH YOUR CHILD ABOUT BIOFEEDBACK

Explain to your child that biofeedback is a tool for learning how to gain control of the nervous system and that it's been proven to help with relaxation and to relieve symptoms for many kinds of pain problems. Because biofeedback often includes wires, sensors, and leads, parents should assure their child that participating in biofeedback will not hurt, nor is there any electricity flowing to the body: biofeedback devices only take information from the body. You can also let your child know that the process is usually fun and interesting.

2. EXPLORE BIOFEEDBACK AT HOME

There are some fun, interactive devices and applications that you and your child can use at home to enhance at-home relaxation practice. Some quality systems include devices made by HeartMath and Wild Divine. These systems typically range in price from $120 to $300. Far less expensive (but also less comprehensive) options include the widely available peripheral thermometers (also called stress thermometers) and biofeedback cards, sometimes referred to as stress cards. There are also a few smartphone applications that can turn a portable phone into a biofeedback device. A portable biofeedback tool may offer children a way to access resources at school or other places, thereby facilitating good coping on the go. If your child has difficulty with biofeedback practice at home, consider that working with a trained biofeedback provider may offer additional benefit. (See opposite page.)

3. FIND A PROVIDER

It's ideal to find a biofeedback provider who has experience working with children. This will help to ensure that the provider will know how to explain the biofeedback equipment and process in a child-friendly and meaningful way. If you are looking for a psychologist, start by asking your child's pediatrician for recommendations, then ask those providers whether they also use biofeedback in their pain-management practice. Alternatively, locate a pain service at the closest major medical center and call them to ask for local providers (see Appendix 4). Despite mounting evidence demonstrating the effectiveness of biofeedback, this service is not covered by most behavioral health insurance

Some recommended biofeedback apps and devices.

Name & Manufacturer	Cost	Description	URL
Bellybio by Relaxline	Free	App for iPhone or iTouch that is placed on the belly to measure movements of the diaphragm while breathing	https://itunes .apple.com/us/app/ bellybio-interactive -breathing/id3537 63955?mt=8
Biofeedback Card sold by iproducts	$2.50–$5.00	Laminated card with temperature-sensitive material that measures peripheral temperature	http://www .products.ws/ biofeedback-cards .html
EMWave2 by HeartMath	$200	Includes software for PC or Mac, and an ear sensor to track heart rhythms	http://store .heartmath.org/ emWave2/ emWave2 -handheld
Inner Balance by HeartMath	$129	Ear sensor is compatible with iPhone/iPads	http://store.heart math.org/Inner -Balance
Relaxing Rhythms by Wild Devine	$300	Includes software and finger sensors that track heart rate and galvanic skin response	http://www.wild divine.com/relaxing -rhythms-software -iom.html
Stress Thermometer sold by Bio-medical	$22	Digital thermom-eter with finger sensor to measure temperature	http://bio-medical .com/products/ stress-thermometer -sc911.html

policies. For this reason, it's generally not possible to use your insurance company to locate a provider. The lack of insurance coverage is one reason why many pain-management specialists integrate biofeedback into a broader practice of pain management, as opposed to offering it as a stand-alone treatment—a comprehensive visit that includes biofeedback is more likely to be covered by insurance.

When locating a provider, it's important to inquire about biofeedback training. Some providers have what is called Biofeedback Certification International Alliance (BCIA) credentials. To identify a provider who is board certified in biofeedback, parents can log on to the BCIA website (www.bcia.org) and look for the "Find a Practitioner" link. Most of these providers are not child specialists, so be sure to find out if an identified provider has experience working with children or adolescents. There are many well-qualified biofeedback providers who have not completed this certification, so parents should remain open to those providers who have experience and training in biofeedback as part of their behavioral medicine training, even if they do not have official biofeedback certifications.

4. PRACTICE IS KEY

Biofeedback is a means to an end. It's a tool that hones and reinforces the active skill of relaxation. It requires practice to become proficient at biofeedback and to have confidence that the techniques are working. If your child is doing biofeedback with a professional, encourage him or her to also practice these relaxation skills at home. If you're using biofeedback tools at home with your child, keep trials short at first so your child does not become frustrated. Parents are also strongly encouraged to try the biofeedback tools themselves. The best way to help your child learn is to successfully demonstrate how to do it yourself, and doing it together will be yet another way you can show your support and encouragement.

Part IV

Go: Getting Kids Going Again

One of the biggest challenges I faced when I first started my career as a pain-management psychologist was figuring out where to start with treatment. When I meet kids they are usually pretty far into a chronic pain problem. This means they are usually struggling regularly with discomfort and are falling behind in school, missing activities, floundering with day-to-day tasks, opting out of social opportunities, and limiting family activities.

Kids and parents come to me with an acute need for relief on all fronts. While it's tempting to jump right in and encourage everyone to restart activities right away, I've learned that this approach runs the risk of alienating my young patients, their parents, or both. Taking a few sessions to explore the foundations of pain management and introducing kids and parents to coping skills fosters the confidence and trust that can lead to a steadier and more meaningful series of successes. And yet even with this ramp-up approach, there can be significant resistance to a new plan to get life back on track. The hardest part is that kids and parents often expect (or hope) that the pain-related symptoms will resolve *before* their child will need to be nudged to return to his or her full and active life. This isn't how the process usually unfolds. Instead, pain-management professionals will typically ask kids to do more even when they are having pain or stress symptoms, because doing more is a big part of how kids can reset their pain alarms and thus start on the path toward feeling better.

Consider the case of Henry, a seventeen-year-old boy with debilitating migraine headaches. He was a junior at a very competitive charter school when I first met him. At the time of his first appointment he had been out of school for five months and was completely isolated from his school, friends, and sport activities. Every day he would have a headache, and almost every evening he would experience escalating, debilitating pain; disruptions to his vision; nausea; and fatigue. He rated his daily pain an "eight out of ten," while his evening pain escalations were off the pain scale and at least once a month required emergency-room interventions. His parents were very supportive of him and had taken him to multiple doctors and systematically helped him to try over a dozen medications. He was continuing to get medical evaluations when I first met him.

Getting Henry and his parents to agree that we needed to pursue getting him back to his usual activities, despite his ongoing symptoms, was tough. Henry was a very bright kid with tremendous academic potential and his parents were understandably distressed that he had "lost" his junior year. As a family, they intuitively worried that his pain would worsen if his life became busier. But after working with Henry and his family to explain the foundations of pain management, and after teaching Henry some coping and relaxation skills, I moved forward with a plan to increase his day-to-day activity levels despite his ongoing and intense pain.

There were three primary challenges with Henry. First, much of Henry's pain was stress-induced and it quickly became clear that any move toward increased function increased his symptoms. Second, Henry was inherently fearful of going out with friends or playing soccer because he worried that his pain would interfere; in other words, social embarrassment and the worry of being sidelined by his pain were inhibiting his progress. And third, Henry's parents had little confidence that he could function in any domain given his persistent and severe symptoms.

Despite these challenges, Henry did make slow and steady progress toward participating more fully in activities that were meaningful to him. His functional recovery was not a quick fix; getting him completely back on track took almost a full year. He completed high school (though he was one full year behind his peers), started playing guitar in a local coffee shop, returned to his soccer team, developed and maintained a romantic relationship, and traveled with his family on a rigorous hiking vacation.

Interestingly, Henry never reported that he felt better. In fact, he continued to report episodes of intense migraine pain and persistent daily headaches. But he continued to make gains. His confidence increased, his social anxiety decreased, and he flourished on many fronts. Because Henry continued to have pain, his parents continued to seek additional remedies and more invasive interventions, but Henry started to decline treatments.

In general, when kids do more every day, we assume they are feeling better. But it's not uncommon for kids like Henry to find a way to be successful and feel better emotionally and functionally even when they continue to report pain. Our goal for all kids is to feel better, but it's important for parents to know that doing more can happen even when symptoms don't appear to resolve and, moreover, that this is a worthwhile goal. Henry always wished his pain would go away, and it was at times very frustrating for him to deal with the challenge of recurrent pain. And yet when Henry was more fully engaged in life, he was happier: he looked forward to living independently and was much more self-assured and confident about his ability to manage his symptoms.

Getting kids back on track is often not an easy task. Yet once parents understand the foundation of chronic pain management, understand what multidisciplinary treatments may support their child's unique pain profile, and have in place the skills and strategies for effectively helping to reset their child's nervous system and increase comfort, they are ready to move forward with getting their child back to a more normal activity level and lifestyle. This is how parents help to restore lasting comfort. This is the "go" part of the plan.

This section of the book, then, is dedicated to the nuts and bolts of how you as a parent can build the scaffolding, or supports, that children need in order to feel that "getting going again" is a positive choice, and one that will lead to success, even if not at first. Chapter 15 provides an overview of how to build an effective behavior plan to guide the process of getting your child back on track. Chapters 16 through 19 detail strategies for how to approach the most common areas of functional difficulties for children with pain, including school, sleep, peers, and family relationships and activities. If your child struggles with all of these domains, rest assured you are in very good company. If your child is functioning well in one or more domains, consider yourself lucky and by all means feel free to skip those chapters, knowing that they're there if you might need them.

In situations where chronic pain and related difficulties are causing minimal impairment, or when there are only one or two areas of function that need attention, a strong parent-child team may be able to make significant gains independently using these strategies. Setting up a plan together to restart the more active or routine parts of life can be a very rewarding experience for parents and their children. Through the process parents and kids learn how to break down difficult problems into smaller, more manageable goals, and to implement useful supports and coping strategies.

Parents should keep in mind, however, that children who have been struggling with chronic pain for a long time and have multiple functional limitations often benefit greatly from working with a behavioral medicine provider. An experienced, caring provider can help create a good behavioral plan, motivate your child to get moving with activities, and keep things on track.

15
Supporting Your Child with Scaffolding

One of the biggest challenges parents face when trying to help support their child's return to function is figuring out when to push their child and when to give him or her a break. My experience with helping many children and families through this process has led me to create some guidelines for thinking about how to systematically make slow and steady gains. Getting a child back on track is a lot like building the scaffolding for a new skyscraper. Just like a construction project, it requires a written blueprint (behavior plan), dedicated crew (family, friends, teachers, doctors), a timeline for progress, and good problem-solving skills in order to address challenges that come up along the way. When we think of scaffolding as the structure that supports the growth of the building, too, it's easy to understand why planning and erecting the scaffolding is such an essential part of the process.

The idea of scaffolding is loosely based on the work of a Russian developmental psychologist named Lev Vygotsky, whose theory on child development emerged in the early 1900s. Vygotsky suggested that a child's optimal development occurs when parents and teachers are able to scaffold a child's learning so that those skills children could do with the help of an adult today they would be able to do independently to-morrow. The goal of the scaffolding is to provide the structure and support a child will need to get back on track. As a general rule, once the scaffolding is in place, parents can feel confident about gently pushing their child forward, knowing that the likelihood for success is high.

The steps for creating this scaffolding are:

1. Identify an area where your child needs to function better in order to be successful (such as school, sleep, sports, helping out at home, and so on).
2. Determine a starting point where you and your child have a high confidence of success.
3. Write up a blueprint for making small, stepwise gains.
4. Document your child's progress.

Now let's consider the key elements that make for successful scaffolding.

Assessing and Building Confidence

Engineers who build skyscrapers have to be highly confident in their designs. Any failures along the way will be costly in terms of time, materials, and expense, so a good plan is essential for building confidence in the project. In a similar way, I think confidence plays a big part in terms of success when we are getting a child back to a normal lifestyle. If kids are continually encouraged to move forward with a plan in which they (or their parents) have low confidence, the risk of failure is greater. In fact, the more times that kids try to get back on track and fail, the more we unintentionally reinforce negative thoughts like "I can't do this" and other feelings of inadequacy, which can undermine future efforts to get kids back on track. So it's important to make sure that a child (and his or her parents) has confidence in any new plan.

Ironically, just when kids need confidence the most, they may feel like they don't have much of it in store. A lack of confidence can be a huge problem for kids who have chronic pain. Many kids feel as if they have failed at playing sports, attending school, hanging out with friends, completing homework, or keeping up with expectations at home. Research shows that when kids perceive themselves as being unsuccessful academically, socially, or athletically, they are more disabled. In other words, feelings of low confidence and low self-efficacy can directly translate into more functional problems. Additionally, fear of pain can lead to low confidence about being able to do even the most basic tasks. For example, a child with foot pain may be afraid of walking even short distances because he fears hurting himself. And if there is a big gap between how a child was previously functioning (or how a child would like to be functioning) and her current ability to get through the day, this chasm can also generate feelings of self-doubt and lead to decreased confidence.

Because low confidence is such a common problem for kids with pain, it's helpful to start with a goal that the child and parents feel can be achieved. And while it may not be reasonable to expect that kids will be 100 percent confident about accomplishing a new goal, as a general guideline I believe kids should be about 80 percent confident that they can succeed. For example, a child who has been out of school for several weeks due to pain may have low confidence in her ability to last through a whole school day. In a situation such as this, school-based accommodations such as adding breaks into the school day, meeting with a school counselor, or being able to participate in an alternate gym class may be part of the scaffolding that helps to increase a child's confidence that he or she can successfully return to school. It's essential to assess a child's confidence level before the plan is implemented. You can do this simply by asking, "On a scale of one to ten, with one being very low confidence and ten being complete confidence, how much confidence do you have that you can successfully stay at school all day?" Let's suppose the child responds with a "three." That's only 30 percent confidence in the plan, which indicates that it will probably not succeed.

So try again with a less ambitious goal: "How much confidence do you have that you can be successful at school until lunch?" Let's suppose the child says "six." We know we are moving in the right direction, but 60 percent confidence is still low. Next you can ask, "How much confidence do you have that you can stay at school from the start of the day until 10 a.m.?" Now let's suppose the child says "eight." That tells us the child has 80 percent confidence that this plan will work. That's pretty good. If a child has high confidence in a plan, he or she is much more likely to be successful with that plan, whatever it might be. I don't generally aim for 100 percent confidence because I recognize that with any challenge there may be some level of self-doubt. A confidence rating of "eight" or "nine" is good enough; we don't need 100 percent confidence to move forward.

As another example, consider the goal of a child's doing more chores around the house. You can break this down into specific chores. Parents can say, "I know it's been hard for you to bend down to empty the dishwasher, but we really need your help around the house. It's important that you do your part. Let's pick a chore for you that requires only a few minutes of your time and energy. I was thinking you could set the table each night for dinner. On a scale of one to ten, how confident are you that you could do this each night?" If your child's confidence is high (eight, nine, or ten), you're all set. If his confidence is low, you can ask how confident he is that he could set the table just four nights per week. If his confidence is still low, you can ask him to pick a chore for which he has higher confidence of success. If you suspect that a low confidence rating is more reflective of an "I don't want to do this at all" sentiment, be clear with your child that doing nothing is not an option. Even if kids aren't jumping at the chance to do more chores, with this framework the conversation that you end up having with your child will be about what he or she *can do* to help out around the house. Doing even a little bit more will jumpstart the process of regaining a healthy activity level, so every small step is worth it.

Making a Blueprint

Every construction project has a blueprint to follow, and likewise, kids need some sort of blueprint in order to follow their plan. Fortunately,

A simple "blueprint" for tracking progress toward goals.

	Mon.	Tues.	Wed.	Thurs.	Fri.	Sat.	Sun.
Goal 1							
Goal 2							

the blueprint for kids can be quite simple. Most plans can be documented on a simple piece of paper that includes a clear and measurable goal, a token reward for success or a consequence for not meeting the goal, and a grid for tracking progress either over the course of a school week, or over a full week. Even in our computer-based world, I've found that writing down the plan on paper, and posting it in a place where parents and kids can both view it, is very effective.

Successful blueprints are simple. They include one or two goals for the week and explicit ways to measure those goals. For example, in the earlier school example, the goal might be to "go to school from 8 a.m. to 10 a.m. every school day." This is a very clear and measurable goal. To make the goal even clearer, if age-appropriate, parents can stipulate that success with this goal means that a child will get dressed each morning without parent prompting. In the chores example, the blueprint goal might state, "Set the table on Monday, Wednesday, Friday, and Sunday." Parents can further stipulate that the table setting must be completed by, say, 5:30 each evening.

We want children to be successful with their goals and to feel good about their progress, so it's very important to track success. Because no one is perfect, I often consider setting up a plan so that a child can be successful if he or she meets approximately 80 percent of the goal for a given time frame. This expectation level allows for some flexibility around unforeseen challenges. Moreover, it provides an opportunity to praise kids for their progress without holding them to a "perfect" standard.

One helpful way to reiterate the idea that a child has to be successful but doesn't have to be perfect is to make an actual "pass card." A pass card can be made on a notecard, sticky note, or folded piece of paper—it doesn't have to be fancy. A child can keep this card and use it when an unforeseen circumstance prevented the attainment of a goal. For example, if the goal is for a child to practice physical therapy exercises seven days per week, but one day he or she just can't fit it into her schedule because there is too much homework, or because she spent the night at a friend's house, she can use her pass card. Even with this one miss, she can still be more than 80 percent successful with her goal. If the goal is to set the table four days a week, one pass card might be given for every two weeks. This would still allow a child to be highly successful, while giving her an opportunity to exert control over the process. If you and your child decide to use a "pass card" as part of the blueprint, you need to be clear about how it can be used. Generally, I like to offer that kids can use the card whenever they want and importantly, that parents can't complain when it's used. If a child hands over a pass card, parents should simply say, "Okay" and move on with the day. No questions asked.

Blueprints can be made for just about any goal, though generally the best goals for a blueprint are those for which there are multiple opportunities for success each week, such as sticking to a home exercise program, taking medication, working on homework for a certain amount of time, completing chores, practicing coping or relaxation strategies, going for a daily walk, eating meals with the family, spending time on a hobby, or taking care of a pet.

When the construction crews of a skyscraper do not adhere to the blueprint, little progress is made. Likewise, if kids and parents do not systematically follow their blueprint, it's hard to attain forward momentum. Parents are usually excited to get moving with a thoughtful and structured plan; kids, however, are prone to drag their feet a bit. Holding kids accountable to the blueprint is an important part of your job as a support person. To help kids in my practice get on board, I like to start a new goal by offering the encouragement of a small reward. Even a small reward can have a big impact, since it's not so much the reward itself that is the incentive, but rather the acknowledgment of a job well done and the hard work involved. My favorite types of rewards are attention-based. For a child who sets the table four nights per week, for example, the reward might be an after-dinner game with Mom or Dad. Alternatively, a reward could be more of a token of appreciation such as a special dessert at the end of the week. Rewards should be small and, importantly, they should be able to be given at the time when the child attains success. This means that a reward such as having a friend sleep over in three weeks is too far from the actual accomplishment to be motivational. Keep rewards small, simple, and expeditious.

On the flip side of the rewards spectrum is the concept of consequences for failure to adhere to a plan. When considering the use of a consequence, I like to remind parents that if the blueprint has been set up right, the goals they have chosen with their child will be small and manageable. In fact, having a good blueprint supported by a system of small, positive rewards is sufficient for many children. If a child fails to jump on board, however, sometimes adding a few "teeth" to the plan can be very effective. To keep it simple, my go-to consequence is the restriction of screen time (time watching TV or playing on a computer, smartphone, or tablet). Yes, adolescents universally cringe at this concept, and that's precisely why it's effective. As with the rewards, the consequence needs to be small and swift. For example, if attending school daily is a goal, failure to attend school on any morning should result in a loss of screen time immediately and just for that day. A failure to set the table four out of seven nights might result in a loss of screen time for twenty-four hours. The actual length of a screen time consequence can be short, even though loss of screen time (for any length of time) will feel like a big deal to most kids.

Limiting screen time can be a little tough on parents as well as kids. For example, it can involve removing TVs or computers from a child's bedroom, or physically confiscating a phone. But it does tend to work well as a motivational tool. And there is another upside to using restricted screen time as a consequence: when kids are not following a plan to increase their mobility and participation in activities, we want to be sure that they are not rewarded in some other way. In other words, a child who stays home from school should not have the privilege of using screens for entertainment. Screens are inherently rewarding, and it would be counterproductive for your child if she felt that staying home from school would be in any way more rewarding than going to school (see Chapter 16 for more on secondary gains).

Of course, other consequences can be equally as effective, and as a parent you should decide what type of consequence, if any, is appropriate for your child. One word of caution: if you do set a consequence, don't cave for any reason. If you set a consequence and your child does not hold up his or her part of the plan, then you simply have to follow through. If you don't follow through, your child gets a strong message—whether you meant to give it or not—that sticking to the blueprint doesn't matter at all. Basically, when parents fail to follow through, kids see no reason to follow through either.

One of the more subtle but very powerful advantages to a clear and effective consequence is that it clearly communicates that regardless of pain, a child can and should be held accountable. Moreover, when parents are unwavering about a consequence, it communicates that kids with pain are not too fragile. We want kids to learn through their experiences that they can do more. Holding kids accountable for not making progress toward an appropriate goal sends that important message.

Blueprints form the foundation of how your child can start to return to a more normal range of activities. Take time to design the blueprint carefully; be sure that you and your child agree and have confidence in the goals. Don't forget to talk with your child about rewards for a job well done, and the possible consequence that comes from failure to adhere to the plan. Once these blueprints are in place, you are off and running. The next step will be to keep the project moving forward.

The Project Timeline

A skyscraper isn't built in a single day; rather, each day the project moves closer to completion. At times progress may be fast and efficient and at other times, for any number of reasons, progress may be slower. While there may be some inherent variability, the overall pacing of the project is important. Keeping a steady pace is the ideal.

With kids who have chronic pain, we use the same approach. It's best to set a steady pace to avoid moving too slowly and to make sure that your child will not lose momentum and fall further behind. And like any big project, it's important to recognize that even when minor setbacks happen, the project continues to move forward.

At the same time it's also important not to move too quickly and overshoot predefined goals. Sometimes an initial feeling of success with a new plan can be so invigorating to kids (and their parents) that they try to push forward quickly to make up for lost time. But this can lead to significant setbacks. For example, if a child feels good at school after attending for two hours a day for one week, he or she may feel ready to attend full days of school the next week. If after trying it he becomes too fatigued or stressed or has too much pain to continue, however, he may end up missing school altogether and lose confidence in the whole plan. It's much better for your child and family if the recovery happens one step at a time, as planned on your blueprint. And if you keep your focus on maintaining forward momentum rather than overemphasizing the end result, you will be less tempted to overshoot.

I think that parents can trust their intuition here. Some kids, especially younger kids who haven't had chronic pain for too long, seem to rebound fairly quickly. I recall working with a seven-year-old girl who was experiencing persistent ankle pain after a surgical repair of a shattered ankle. She was fearful and reported that she was in too much pain to stop using crutches. The challenge was that her physician and physical therapist felt she no longer needed crutches and wanted her to walk again without support. In session, we set up a blueprint to help increase her confidence and stamina for walking without the use of crutches. After a thorough discussion during which we assessed her confidence level, we determined that she had high confidence she could take seven steps without crutches, and she agreed to do this three times a day for one week. She was given two pass cards for the week and her reward was to get a new bottle of nail polish to paint her toenails. In the first week she accomplished her goals and felt very proud of herself. In our next session she came in (with toenails painted) and a very positive attitude. I'd intended to increase her walking without crutches slowly, and suggested that she try taking fourteen steps three times per day. But both she and her Mom had confidence that she could do more. In a private discussion with her Mom, I learned that for this child, fear of pain was the biggest problem. Her Mom shared that her accomplishments this week had really helped to reduce that fear and to increase her confidence. So we all decided to have her stop using crutches at home and to go for a ten-minute walk outside each day without crutches. When I saw her the following week she was beaming. She had followed the plan for the first four days of the week and then decided she was feeling much, much better and didn't need her crutches at all. They were actually late for their appointment because she had been out riding her bike that afternoon. Importantly, in this case, the child was medically cleared for full activity. Her stalled progress in terms of regaining her function for walking was almost entirely due to her fear of pain and low confidence. She and her Mom both knew that she was ready to move forward quickly and doing so worked out very well for her.

While a more rapid recovery like this is sometimes possible, it's certainly not typical. In my experience, setting the bar for success too high more often triggers increased pain, frustration, and disability. Maintaining stepwise and steady progress should be the default setting for the vast majority of blueprints. This may require that parents stop rushing and temporarily let go of their own fears and anxieties about their child falling behind in school, missing athletic practice, or losing contact with friends. When parents take a step back and assess their child's suffering, which can include a combination of pain, anxiety, fear, sadness, and other factors, they can often get a sense of the complexity involved with getting back on track. As a general rule, the longer pain has been around, the longer it can take to get a child back to a more typical schedule of activities. The temptation to speed through the recovery efforts can overwhelm kids and disrupt their progress.

◆

How to Help

1. BE EXPLICIT

Talk openly to your child about the need to get back to all of the fun parts of life, and to rejoin friends and family in a more active way. Explain the scaffolding approach by saying that you will put good supports in place and that your child will move slowly and steadily toward goals you decide on together by following a blueprint, or plan. Be sure to emphasize that your child will be involved in making the plan and that both you and your child need to have confidence in the goals.

2. IDENTIFY A GOAL (OR TWO) TO WORK ON FIRST

Work together with your child to identify one or two goals to target at a time. For example, a child might work on school and exercise. Or a child might set goals for sleeping more regularly and participating in social activities. In choosing a goal, be sure to work with your child to find one that is challenging, but attainable. Use the confidence question ("On a scale of one to ten, how confident are you that you can be successful with . . . ?") to ensure that before you jump in to work on a goal, your child has reasonably high confidence that he or she can achieve it. Once you make progress with one or two goals, you can expand your blueprint to include others.

3. MAKE A BLUEPRINT

Make a simple grid that includes the goal or goals, clear rewards and/ or consequences, and the days of the week so you and your child can track progress. The goals should be as clear and specific as possible.

For example, instead of "go for a walk every day," try "walk for six blocks" or "walk for twelve minutes." Similarly, instead of "be more relaxed," you might use "practice guided imagery for fifteen minutes." As part of the blueprint, consider making one or two "pass cards" with your child. Grab a piece of paper or notecard, write "pass card" on it, and give it to your child. Kids can then use the pass whenever they want to opt out of a goal for just that one time, without consequences. Parents will then have to do their part by graciously accepting the pass when it is presented.

4. DEVELOP A PROJECT TIMELINE

As a general rule of thumb, think about moving forward in increments of 10 to 30 percent; that is, each week you and your child should aim to increase the activity level or amount of time participating in an outside activity by 10 to 30 percent. Remember that making progress is a matter of balance: if your child doesn't keep making some forward progress, he or she may lose momentum with the entire plan, but making gains too quickly risks future setbacks. Keep in mind that in general, the longer your child has had functional difficulties, the longer it may take her to regain her full function. Even so, parents should expect that their child will follow through with the plan, even in the context of discomfort or pain. This may be difficult for everyone involved, but parents should take comfort in knowing that this will help their child learn that she can manage pain symptoms and still have a full and enjoyable life.

5. CONSIDER SETTING REWARDS AND/OR CONSEQUENCES

My general feeling about rewards is that they can be very helpful for reinforcing successes and helping children feel as though their efforts are paying off. My favorite rewards include small things like making a child's favorite dinner, allowing a child to earn a special privilege, or, best of all, giving a child one-on-one attention that is not focused on pain or recovery efforts. I urge parents to steer clear of monetary rewards, material gifts that exceed a few dollars, or activities that are difficult to schedule. Rewards are most reinforcing when they are given at the time of success, so if you have identified a reward with your child, be sure you are prepared to give it just as soon as your child accomplishes that goal. Consequences, if used, should also be small and, to be effective, need to be meaningful to your child. Loss of screen time is an easy, effective consequence with the positive benefit of making staying at home less appealing, but remember that the length of time should be short and predefined. If you do assign a consequence, follow-through is critical.

6. CONSULT WITH OTHERS

If you are working with a behavioral medicine provider, developing a blueprint for increased function can be an integrated part of your child's care. If not, you the parent will need to check with your child's physicians, physical therapists, schools, and so on to ensure that the goals will work within the scope of a child's overarching medical plan and in the context of these other important commitments.

7. REMEMBER, SKYSCRAPERS AREN'T BUILT IN A DAY

If your child does not achieve a goal, don't give up. Recognize the progress your child did make and the effort involved. Discuss where modifications are needed, make those adjustments, and try again. As any good architect at the helm of a skyscraper construction project might tell you, a stalled project can indicate the need for additional workers or resources. Don't hesitate to reach out for additional supports to help in your important work of getting your child back on track.

16

A Balanced Approach to the Problem of School

Research shows that more than 50 percent of kids with pain have trouble keeping up with the demands of school. Disruptions include repeated absences, difficulty completing homework on time, lower grades, and an increased risk for being bullied at school. On average, kids with pain miss four to five days of school per month, with those children experiencing high levels of pain missing substantially more. More than 40 percent of parents report that pain has interfered with their child's academic performance, even though in many cases kids with pain are likely to be conscientious students who are perceived by teachers as being better adjusted than their peers.

When children are out of school for even a short period of time, they feel overwhelmed with make-up work, out of step with the current social scene, and disconnected from the classroom environment. For all children, there is an inherent level of stress associated with the school day: waking up early, academic pressure, and social challenges are among the most common problems. But for children with pain, these problems can be magnified. Additionally, research shows that when a child's nervous system is stuck in a chronic pain cycle, he or she may temporarily have more difficulty with concentration, learning, and memory—perhaps as a direct result of the nervous system's response to pain. Difficulty with memory and concentration can also be related to numerous types of pain medications, disrupted sleep, and anxiety or mood-related symptoms that may co-occur with chronic pain. This disruption to typical thinking and memory patterns can make concentration on schoolwork a very big challenge. For all of these reasons, many children feel that attending school is often too difficult. While school stress is significant for children with chronic pain, staying out of school only tends to make the problem much, much worse.

I won't sugarcoat this. Getting back on track at school is often extremely difficult for kids with pain, especially if they have been out of school for six weeks or more. Many children are resistant to efforts to increase their time or performance at school, at least initially, and this resistance can take the form of openly refusing to go to school, refusing to agree to a school plan, or agreeing to a school plan and then finding reason after reason that the plan can't work. Resistance to school may be because, given their pain, children may not feel they can be successful at learning the academic material, hanging out with friends, or even simply sitting through their school day. Getting back on track at school is also extremely difficult for parents; it takes a lot of time, energy, diplomacy, and persistence. Staying focused on the idea that getting back to school helps a child's pain problem is paramount to success. Learning how to help build a child's school-based confidence from the inside out is one of the primary objectives.

I get one of three reactions from parents when the topic of school comes up. If parents have not yet heard that getting back to school is an early goal for pain recovery, they tend to look at me wide-eyed as if to say, "Do you see how much pain my child is in? I can't believe you're talking about getting back on track at school." In contrast to this, some parents have already heard from multiple other providers that they need to get their child back to school sooner rather than later. These parents will often nod agreeably when I talk about it. Even so, over the years I've learned that many of these agreeable parents may only be nodding to be polite. Of course they want their child back in school and realize that it's an important goal, but these parents may lack the confidence that now is the right time to take the plunge. And then there is the third group of parents. These are the parents that are in fact ready to take the plunge. These parents understand the foundational principles of pain management and feel confident that their child has some tools in place to foster comfort. They desperately want to get their child back in full swing as far as school is concerned and they know that there is no time like the present to get started, even if they don't know yet how to do it effectively. Wherever you are in thinking about your child's school attendance and performance, rest assured you are in good company. Importantly, there are ideas and strategies within this chapter that can help to prepare you and your child for increased school success at any stage of readiness.

Why Is Your Child Struggling with School?

Before coming up with the scaffolding and blueprint to support your child, you have to understand *why* your child is struggling on the school front. All children with pain report that pain is the underlying reason that they are not in school or that grades have suffered. But there are many reasons why children struggle with school, and often there is more than one reason that children with pain are either not attending school or are underperforming while there. When we dig a little deeper, we often find that other factors such as social anxiety, performance anxiety, learning disabilities, low self-esteem, peer-based stress, bullying, or wishes for parental attention or other rewards outside of school are perpetuating school-based struggles. Before you can make an effective plan, you need to figure out what's going on.

Start by talking in a general way with your child about the hardest part of school. Is your child worried about poor grades, feeling disconnected from friends, being teased, feeling lost or confused in class, feeling unsure about how to talk with friends about their pain problem, concerned about leaving home, or has he or she lost the motivation to attend? All of these school-based problems are common, but of course none of these actually mean that a child should stay out of school.

Having empathy, patiently asking questions and listening in a non-judgmental way to any answers your child gives are very important when you discuss these challenges. Take your time with this step. Give your child the emotional space to talk about all the facets of school that pose difficulty. Here are some of the phrases you may hear your child say during this important conversation.

"I'M LOST."

Being out of school creates an enormous amount of stress. Being lost can relate to feeling out of touch with the school routine or feeling confused and overwhelmed by the schoolwork. In high school where all grades seem to be viewed in the context of impending college applications, and the complexity and volume of work are dramatically greater than in middle or elementary school, being "lost" can be especially terrifying. Feeling "lost" is an inevitable part of being out of school, and even kids who work hard at home to catch up express having that sensation for several days or weeks after they return to school.

"I FEEL BETTER AT HOME."

"Secondary gain" is the technical term that is used to describe the benefits that children receive when they stay home. Such benefits might include staying up late and sleeping late; unlimited TV, computer, or video time; extra one-on-one time with a parent; extra treats or attention; or hanging out all day in pajamas. Such a pile-up of subtle and not-so-subtle incentives is a common problem when children have been out of school for a while. Secondary gains may not be what originally created the concerns about school, but they can perpetuate it. Parents need to be aware that even if their child claims to want to be in school, being at home can unintentionally be very rewarding. The treatment for secondary gain is to make staying home during the day *less* rewarding, at least until the going to school part of your child's life is back on track. Parents have to develop stringent rules for what happens if their child absolutely cannot attend school. These rules should include set times for waking up, getting dressed, and meals; restricted time on all screens (TVs, smartphones, computers, video games, and tablets); and a designated time for homework or make-up work.

"I CAN'T MAKE IT THROUGH A WHOLE SCHOOL DAY."

Many kids with chronic pain struggle to get through the physical demands of a full school day. Sitting all day in hard chairs, paying attention in class, having to answer questions and take tests, having limited access to bathrooms, carrying heavy backpacks, and other factors can all be difficult for a child in pain. Moreover, each time that kids try and fail, they reinforce their belief that they can't make it through the day. The key here is to have your child rack up successes. By slowly increasing the time each week that your child will go to school, and ensuring that he or she has the appropriate accommodations in place to address specific barriers or challenges while at school, your child should be able to make steady progress.

"I JUST CAN'T GET GOING IN THE MORNING."

Many kids with pain feel their worst when they wake up in the morning. Muscles may be tight or achy, children with irritable bowel syndrome or functional abdominal pain may have more gastrointestinal upset, headaches can be significant, and persistent fatigue from disrupted sleep all combine to make mornings a tough time of day. When kids wake up in the morning and the whole long school day looms in front of them, it's a hard sell to get them out the door. But once kids do get out the door and into school, and the distractions and fun parts of the school day get going, many kids can rally and succeed. I usually advocate for kids to get out the door in the morning and start the school day with their peers even if they hurt or are not at their best. Sometimes, however, such as when you're just starting out on your blueprint and helping your child get back into the swing of school with a limited school day, it can be helpful to give your child some say as to what time of day he or she will attend.

Remember, approximately one in four children will experience an episode of chronic pain in his or her lifetime. That means that within any given classroom, chances are high that other students have had a chronic pain-related experience. But your child may still feel misunderstood, since despite the frequency with which this situation occurs, school personnel are frequently in the dark about chronic pain issues and how to support kids. Similarly, peers are often not sure how to respond. You can help. Meet with your child's teachers and principal to be sure that the staff and faculty working with your child are knowledgeable about chronic pain. It's also essential to ensure that your child knows how to advocate for himself or herself at school and how to respond to peers (for more advice on this, see Chapter 18).

Once you talk with your child about the most daunting challenge or challenges on the school front, you can move forward and make a plan together to address these difficulties. For example, if your child has been out of school for several weeks and feels lost, a slow reentry into school that combines exposure in the classroom with extra after-school teacher support may help to target the issue. If peer-based difficulties are the concern, meeting with school guidance counselors and helping your child to foster new friendships either in or outside of school may be important goals. If sitting all day in class is the primary challenge, you might want to ask whether a different seat or planned breaks could be arranged. As a parent, you don't have to have all the answers to the challenges; you just need to understand what the primary challenges are and be willing to brainstorm with your child and the school staff about how to address the issues at hand.

Collaborating with School Staff

After developing a list of challenges and perhaps brainstorming some ideas to address these challenges with your child, the next step is to get the school staff involved. Many schools welcome collaboration with parents and are eager to try to increase a child's attendance and performance. These schools may also ask to talk to the medical team working with your child and have staff willing to learn new approaches to help a child with a chronic pain problem. The first step is yours. Call the school and let them know that you're concerned about your child's ability to succeed in school. Request a meeting with your child's teachers (as many as possible) and guidance staff about your child's school attendance or performance. For younger children, the meeting should include your child's primary teacher, a school nurse, a school counselor (if available), and a head of school (principal, assistant principal). For high school students, the meeting should include a guidance counselor, school nurse, a head of school, and teachers. It can sometimes be best if your child does not go to the initial school meeting, so that you and the school staff can talk openly about potential barriers or past problems without increasing your child's stress. It is important, however, to have your child present at any meetings when new plans or accommodations will be discussed.

Deirdre Logan, my colleague at the Pain Treatment Service, has found in her research that teachers are more likely to support students with pain when they have access to a doctor's note that includes documentation or explanation of a child's condition and a list of a child's current medical and school-based challenges. Moreover, teachers are more receptive to supporting a child when they perceive that the parents are working cooperatively with them to help address concerns. For these reasons, parents should arrive at a school meeting prepared to educate staff about their child's pain problem and to provide teachers and school personnel with permission to contact the medical professionals who are working with their child. This willingness to include your child's pain management professionals will foster a trusting and collaborative interdisciplinary approach to managing chronic pain at school.

During the meeting, be sure to discuss how your child's pain influences her school performance or attendance. Challenges that accompany chronic pain may range from physical limitations—like not being able to walk up stairs, pain from carrying a heavy backpack, an inability to write, or the need to use the bathroom frequently—to environmental sensitivities such as not being able to tolerate noise in the lunchroom, preference for alternate seating or the use of a seat cushion, or needing to sit close to the teacher to stay on track.

Parents may also want to discuss school-based triggers for their child's pain. For example, if your child's pain is triggered by hunger, bright lights, or sitting for too long, parents should bring this to the attention of the school. Parents are advised to put all of their concerns in writing along with a list of some preliminary ideas for how to support their child. The meeting should include a discussion about what accommodations are needed and whether they require an official school plan.

During the meeting, parents should remain open to suggestions, be prepared to make compromises, and demonstrate a willingness to give new ideas a try. This mindset is really important. Strive to make the spirit of the meeting open and collaborative, even if there is some resistance to putting in place your family's preferred accommodations. Having a positive approach to the meeting will keep school staff engaged and increase their willingness to address your child's needs.

Parents are encouraged to maximize the time they have with the staff and be proactive in identifying upcoming situations that are anticipated to be difficult (such as field trips or standardized testing days). Hopefully the staff will be interested in brainstorming with you to manage these challenges with specific accommodations. Before the meeting closes, it's important for parents to identify one point person who can be their ongoing contact. Parents should maintain regular phone or email communication to keep this person informed of progress—or setbacks—on all fronts.

Keep in mind that schools vary considerably in their willingness to support a child with chronic pain. When kids have had a lot of absences, or when the school staff members don't fully understand a child's medical condition even after your attempts to help them with this process, there can be tension. Sometimes this results in a school reporting repeated absences as truancies, penalizing a child by not allowing adequate time for make-up work, or communicating with parents in a strained or even hostile way. When parents feel they are not able to work effectively with school personnel or consistently have difficulty communicating with them, it can be enormously useful to enlist the assistance of a psychologist, physician, social worker, or designated school advocate. Parents should not feel pressured to agree to a school plan that does not feel right for their child. If parents find themselves in this situation with school personnel, parents are encouraged to stay pleasant and ask to continue the conversation at a later point. The next meeting can then include a medical or behavioral medicine provider, or a professional school advocate, who can help to bridge the communication gap.

Section 504 Plans and Individualized Education Programs

Some schools are very cooperative and are well prepared to develop individual blueprints or plans to support children with chronic pain and pain-related difficulties. Other schools are less knowledgeable about how to help in these circumstances or may not have adequate resources in place. If your child's school is open to accommodation and is collaborative in its approach to supporting your child, you do not necessarily need to pursue a formalized school accommodation plan, especially if you anticipate that your child will need only short-term accommodations. Instead, it should be enough to have a school meeting and maintain good ongoing communication.

If you experience significant resistance from the school, or if you anticipate that accommodations or services are going to be needed for many months or years, you may need to request a formal school accommodation plan. Within the United States these formal school plans are termed Section 504 plans and individualized education plans (IEPs). These plans vary by state, but some general information about these resources may be useful.

SECTION 504 PLANS

In the United States, Section 504 is the part of the Rehabilitation Act of 1973 that protects children with a disability in educational settings by ensuring that they can have equal access to school-based services. When a child has a physical or mental impairment, whether permanent or temporary, schools are required to make accommodations so the student may participate as fully as possible in the general curriculum. Section 504 plans can be sought for chronic pain, chronic illness, physical disability, and mental health diagnoses, and they allow for resources and environmental accommodations to be put in place to ensure that a child has an appropriate learning environment. The plan is put together in collaboration with parents and school staff and typically requires a note from a physician or mental health provider documenting that the child has a condition that qualifies for the plan. The plans are individually constructed, are typically designed to be flexible to meet a child's changing needs, and can be readily updated or discontinued when services are no longer needed.

INDIVIDUALIZED EDUCATION PROGRAMS

The individualized education program, or IEP, arose from a U.S. federal statute within the Individuals with Disabilities Education Act (IDEA). An IEP is a more comprehensive education plan and is typically reserved for children who have disabilities that significantly affect their educational progress. If your child already has an IEP in place, it can often be modified to accommodate additional needs that relate to chronic pain. If your child does not have an IEP, initiating one usually requires an educational assessment and this can often be done through the school system.

There are pros and cons to Section 504s and IEPs. Both are official documents and school staff are required to adhere to the agreed-on stipulations within the plan. The advantage of the Section 504 is that is can usually be put into place quickly, is easily modified, and can be a useful tool for addressing environmental factors or obtaining additional academic supports. The disadvantage to the Section 504 is that it does not typically cover more comprehensive educational services such as special needs classes or adjunctive school-based therapies such as occupational or physical therapy. Section 504 plans also do not require teachers or support staff to record a child's progress. Indeed, whether the Section 504 plan is succeeding is a subjective decision and the stipulations of the Section 504 plans are reviewed only minimally each year.

Compared to the Section 504 plans, IEPs are much more comprehensive, and the results of changes made under IEPs are more carefully monitored and recorded by school staff. Additionally, in most states IEPs remain in place for three years. The disadvantage to IEPs is that because they are more comprehensive and open the door to many additional services, they are harder to qualify for, can take longer to be put in place, and can be more challenging to modify than a Section 504 plan.

As a general rule, when a child is struggling in school, I often advocate for a Section 504 plan initially. If it becomes clear that a child's needs are more long-term or if learning issues are a primary problem, then we move toward advocating for an IEP.

Accommodation Options

Accommodations vary depending on a child's specific pain problem and school-related difficulties. In general, any school plan should encourage a child to be as active and functional as possible at school. For example, if a child can walk with crutches, avoid advocating for the use of a wheelchair in school. Instead, ask for accommodations that will help to make your child comfortable using crutches while at school (for example, your child may need to leave class a few minutes early to avoid crowded hallways or have a friend carry her books at times).

Below is a list of possible accommodations. You should pick only those accommodations that will be instrumental in addressing your child's specific problem. For example, if your child has headaches, you probably won't need special transportation. If buses are noisy and that causes headache pain, your child can use other creative solutions such as earplugs or listening to music. Keep in mind that many of these accommodations, especially those that stipulate for reduced attendance, are viewed as temporary measures to support a child's return to school. After attaining the increased confidence and success that come from getting back to school for a shorter day or using other accommodations, most kids are typically expected to ease back into a full school schedule.

Accommodations by the school may include allowing your child to:

Start the school day late
Leave school early
Take fewer classes
Receive extra time on assignments
Receive fewer or smaller assignments
Take alternate transportation
Obtain a second set of books to keep at home
Have in-school academic or tutoring support
Be assigned a note-taking buddy
Have access to the teacher's notes
Receive home-based tutoring
Participate in physical or occupational therapy
Sit in a special place in the classroom
Receive support from the school nurse
Leave the classroom as needed
Have unrestricted use of the bathrooms
Have access to an elevator instead of stairs
Contact a parent for pick-up
Go to the library or nurses office for relaxation
Eat lunch in a quiet place
Receive counseling or social support
Take courses pass/fail

All school plans need to be flexible and may change over time. When kids have been out of school for weeks or months, the plans should start with more accommodation to ensure that kids and parents feel supported in achieving the initial goals. The point is to boost your child's confidence during the first days and weeks back at school, so that he realizes that he can function even if pain is ongoing.

Visiting the School Nurse

Remember the pass-card system from Chapter 15? That same approach can be used to give a child a break during the school day. Nurses can be great allies when working with the school. Not only can they understand and interpret medical reports for other staff and assist with medications as needed, they also can help kids to get a much-needed reprieve in the middle of a busy or stressful school day. Parents would be wise to meet with the school nurse and patiently explain their child's situation, so that the school nurse will be sympathetic to their child's needs. If your child is hesitant to go to the nurse because she worries the nurse won't understand her pain, arrange for you both to meet with the nurse to get this relationship off to a strong start.

As a general rule, I suggest that kids with pain or pain-related stress arrange to be able to go to the school nurse one to three times per day. For this to work, the school nurse and teachers need to be informed and on board, and of course, the number of visits depends on how many hours a day a child is in school and how severe the pain is. For example, if a child has significant pain and is in school all day, he or she may need a brief break every two to three hours. If the pain is mild, or if a child is temporarily attending only a partial day of school, however, fewer breaks will be needed.

As with passes at home, a school pass card can be as simple as a notecard or folded piece of paper. When a pass-card system is used for school breaks, kids should be given the designated number of passes each day. Each pass card can be worth a fifteen-minute break. During a pass-card break, a child might rest quietly in a cot or chair, listen to music or a relaxation exercise with earbuds, or practice a relaxation exercise such as deep breathing or progressive muscle relaxation. At the end of fifteen minutes, the child should return to class.

A plan like this ensures that a child can remain at school for longer periods of time while still feeling like there is a way to find relief from his or her pain. When nurses get on board with this plan, they frequently welcome kids into the office because they know the children will be there for only fifteen minutes and they won't have to negotiate a return to class or report to the parents every time. When kids understand the plan, too, they feel less awkward about going to the nurse, more relaxed knowing that they can have a break in the day if needed, and supported because they know that they can talk to a parent if they are still experiencing strong pain after using up all of their passes. For all of these reasons, setting the expectation that a child can take a preset number of breaks in the day can really help, especially for kids who are reluctant to actively seek support in school.

For those children who rather enjoy visiting the nurse at school, pass cards can also be a useful tool. First assess approximately how many times per day a child is going to the nurse's office. Then plan to slowly decrease the number of visits and the length of each visit by reducing the number of passes issued each day and shortening the time allowed for each pass. It's important to go slowly so your child feels confident that he or she can be successful in limiting visits to the nurse. If your child is going to the nurse's office seven times in a day, for example, you might reduce that to six passes per day for a few days. That means that your child can go to the nurse six times and stay for fifteen minutes each time. She is entitled to use all six passes, but when the passes are used up, she must remain in the classroom for the rest of the day. Interestingly, when kids are in control of the passes, they tend to save them and go less often to the nurse, just in case they may need the passes later in the day. If your child starts with six passes for a few days, you can then reduce the number to five passes, and then four passes. Once you get down to three passes, you can stay at that number. In most cases, kids with pain should be entitled to keep at least a few passes with them so they feel they always have nurse access if needed. If your child needs more of an incentive to cooperate with this plan, you can offer small rewards for a successful week with an added bonus to cash in all unused passes for the week. For example, if your child uses only four of her six allotted passes, she can cash in the two extra passes for two chocolate kisses or another token reward.

Ongoing Advocacy and Diplomacy

Parents should anticipate frequent bumps in the road to developing an effective school plan and be ready to roll with the challenges. Part of "rolling with it" is to stay positive and refrain from telling their child that, for example, they were frustrated at a school meeting or teachers were not as flexible or accommodating as hoped. Sharing this information only serves to increase a child's stress. Moreover, if parents become bitter or angry with the school, their children may act that way as well. Instead, parents should send the message to their child that they are confident that a good school plan can be devised. When parents model a collaborative and problem-solving relationship with school staff, their child is far more likely to adopt that same approach.

It's vitally important for parents to be a strong advocate for their child, but it is equally important to teach and encourage children to advocate on their own behalf. Early in the process of setting up a school plan, parents need to set the expectation that their child will help to address minor problems and learn to ask for help when needed. While parents are essential for helping to negotiate or manage any big problems that arise, they should avoid micro-managing their child's school situation.

Remember, too, to pay compliments when they are due. Of course parents and children should let school providers know if a plan is not working so issues can be appropriately addressed. But it is equally important for parents and kids to tell the school staff when a new plan or accommodation is working well. This positive feedback can go a long way toward fostering a lasting positive and collaborative relationship with the school.

What about Home-Based Programs?

Some parents conclude that traditional school settings are just not right for their child and begin to investigate educational programs outside the traditional school setting. Home-based programs can take the form of full-time home-based tutoring support in cooperation with a public school, online education, parent-led education, or home-schooling consortiums.

I recognize that the idea of a home-based education is never tossed around lightly. By the time parents conclude that their child needs to be educated at home, they have often tried numerous accommodations at school and feel that their child has either lost too much time at school to make reentry a worthwhile endeavor academically, or that their child just can't negotiate the inherent challenges in the school setting.

While home-schooling can seem like the next best option in this situation, as a general rule I strongly caution against this step. Home-based education may seem to relieve many school-based challenges including the need to wake up early, negotiate peer relationships, and manage difficult classes. But the long-term losses tend to outweigh the short-term gains. Beyond the educational merits, being involved in a typical school setting means children have daily opportunities for peer interactions, get in the routine of functioning independently from parents, and importantly are able to practice accountability in the context of pain, a skill that serves children well beyond their medical challenges. For all of these reasons, I routinely recommend that kids with pain should stay connected and involved in a traditional school setting.

Currently there is no research evidence that addresses the long-term outcomes of home-based schooling for children with pain. Providers who have been in the field for a long time, however, have noticed a trend. Charles Berde, founder and chief of our Pain Treatment Service, has treated thousands of children with chronic pain as well as those in need of palliative care. In his experience, children who are home-schooled due to pain or pain-related stress become increasingly isolated, demonstrate more pain and disability, and have greater dependence on parents, all of which moves them further away from their long-term goals of living a full and independent life.

Within my clinical practice, on a few rare occasions, I've seen how a partial or full year of home-schooling has provided the flexibility necessary for a child to fully attend to their rehabilitation needs. But for a child who has been home-schooled, reintegration into a typical school setting can be very challenging. In fact, when the time comes to rejoin the school community, I recommend that a behavioral medicine provider be enlisted to help solve any problems that may arise along the way.

Could My Child Have a Learning Difficulty?

Many types of learning disability do not show up at an early age and may only be apparent when the complexity of a child's work increases. For example, transitions to junior high and high school are times when underlying learning difficulties may become obvious. Parents should especially take notice if their child has a growing discrepancy between grades in a favorite subject and non-favorite subject, a history of learning difficulty such as a delay in learning to read, or persistent struggles with organization or memory. Parents should also take notice of potential red flags such as a child frequently complaining that the work is too hard or that bad teachers are routinely the cause of low grades. Other red flags can be a child becoming overwhelmed by big projects or assignments or frequently using avoidance-based strategies that lead to struggles over homework. If you are concerned about your child's learning, don't hesitate to request an educational or neuropsychological evaluation either through the school system or through a private neuropsychologist.

The Case of Amanda

Amanda was thirteen years old and finishing eighth grade when her abdominal pain started. It didn't interfere much with school, and she had a good summer with few episodes of pain. She looked forward to starting her freshman year in high school along with her many girlfriends, and the first few weeks of school seemed to go very well both socially and academically. By the end of October, however, Amanda was experiencing one to three episodes of debilitating abdominal pain per week. On the days when she had bad pain she struggled to wake up in the morning and pleaded with her parents to stay home. If the abdominal pain came on while she was at school, she spent much of her day in the nurse's office or in the bathroom. When she got home from school, Amanda often fell asleep on the couch and refused to do homework. By November, Amanda was routinely missing three days of school a week. She also had at least one morning a week when she went to school late. She had been evaluated by physicians and diagnosed with functional abdominal pain. Her medical team strongly encouraged a return to school and increased function as part of her treatment plan.

Amanda and her parents argued every morning about whether or not she felt well enough to go to school, and her parents were increasingly frustrated with her refusals to go because she was rapidly falling behind in all of her classes. Indeed, her parents were becoming very concerned with her mounting pile of make-up work and were angry with the school staff for what they perceived to be a lack of initiative to help Amanda. The more school that Amanda missed, the more she didn't want to go to school; unsympathetic teachers and inquiring peers made her increasingly uncomfortable there. Additionally, she worried that she would have a pain episode at school and be unable to manage her symptoms.

The first step was to understand *why* Amanda was missing school. Abdominal pain along with feeling uncomfortable talking to teachers and peers were the main issues. Academically Amanda was doing well, but the imposing pile of make-up work was also daunting for her. The goals for Amanda, then, were to (1) increase her attendance at school, (2) increase the time she spent doing homework, and (3) reduce her social anxiety while at school.

MEETING WITH SCHOOL STAFF

Amanda's parents notified the school staff that they needed to meet to discuss a behavioral plan for Amanda and requested that a guidance counselor, Amanda's teachers, and a principal or assistant principal be present. Amanda's parents took to the meeting documentation from Amanda's doctors to show that she had been evaluated for her abdominal pain and that she was cleared to attend school but would need some accommodations. They discussed Amanda's attendance difficulties, make-up homework, ongoing pain, as well as the fact that she was feeling nervous about talking to kids and teachers in school.

At the meeting, the group made an appointment for Amanda to meet with the guidance counselor to discuss the social anxiety she was experiencing. And together, Amanda's parents and school staff came up with the following list of accommodations:

Permission to leave school early without penalty
Extra time to complete assignments
Reduced assignments (to decrease the volume of make-up work)
Access to the school nurse (via a pass system)
Access to bathrooms as needed
Permission to call home if her pain persisted past 11:00 a.m.
In-school tutoring support on Friday afternoons
Weekly meetings with the guidance counselor to address peer anxiety
Teachers would be alerted to her anxiety and kindly requested not to single her out in class about her absences

The school was eager to have the family pursue a formal Section 504 education plan and reported that they would incorporate these accommodations into her plan. Moreover, they agreed to share information about Amanda's abdominal pain with all of Amanda's teachers so that Amanda wouldn't have to explain the situation to them. Amanda's parents discussed their goals of slowly increasing Amanda's attendance and homework time over the next few weeks, and they were told to contact the vice principal with any questions, concerns, or updates.

CONSTRUCTING THE BLUEPRINT

The next step was to create a blueprint for making progress on Amanda's functional goals of attending school more regularly and spending longer on homework. To find a starting point, Amanda's parents checked in with her about her confidence level. When they started making the plan, Amanda was going to school on average only two mornings per week. She was highly doubtful that she could make it through a full day of school, but felt confident that she could manage one more morning each week. Amanda and her parents decided that she had to stay at school until 11:00 a.m. to qualify for a successful morning. Her goal for her first week, then, was to attend school from 8:00–11:00 a.m. on Monday, Wednesday, and Friday.

For the goal of increasing homework time, Amanda had to start very small. At the time that her parents started her blueprint, Amanda was refusing to do all homework and was unsure how much she could accomplish. She and her parents thus settled on a goal of eight minutes of homework each night. Even though this goal seems too small to make a difference in her big pile of work, it was still a way to set out in the right direction. Amanda's blueprint was intended to boost her confidence and fuel continued success.

PUTTING THE PLAN INTO ACTION

At home, Amanda and her parents came up with a reward and consequence for her school blueprint. Each Friday night, if Amanda had been successful with her attendance goal, she earned a movie night at home with her parents. If she had been successful with her homework goal for the week, she earned a new song for her iPhone. And if she didn't complete her attendance and homework goals for the week, there were consequences. She lost all screen time for the weekend if she missed her attendance goals for the week. Amanda's parents typically allowed her to have one hour of screen time each weekday night, but as part of this plan she was not permitted to have any screen time until she completed her eight minutes of homework. If she missed her homework goal for a night, as a consequence, she would lose her screen-time privilege entirely for that evening.

To give Amanda some autonomy in the blueprint, Amanda was given one pass card for the week to use at home if she needed a night off of her homework goal due to pain, fatigue, or other reasons. And on the school front, Amanda was given one pass card daily to use at school if she needed to visit the nurse for a break between 8:00 and 11:00 a.m. All of the teachers were told that she could leave the classroom as needed to use the bathroom. Wednesday mornings she would meet with the school psychologist to address social concerns. And every Friday after her 11:00 a.m. dismissal, she would return to school at 3:00 p.m. for tutoring support.

The chart for week 1 shows a very successful week for Amanda. She fully met her attendance goals. This means that instead of feeling sad and disappointed and battling about school attendance, Amanda and her parents felt very positive about her efforts. Additionally, she completed eight minutes of homework four nights per week. She used her pass card on the first night, but still met her goal. Because she met both of her assigned goals, she and her parents could celebrate with praise, her movie reward, and a new song for her iPhone. Additionally, Amanda's parents told the teachers and the other staff whom they were coordinating with at school that Amanda had met her attendance and homework goals for her first week. While there was still much work to be done, it was useful for the school staff to know that things were moving in the right direction and thoughtful for her parents to share the good news with them.

Amanda's first week.

School attendance blueprint:

Goal	Go to school Monday, Wednesday, and Friday until 11:00 a.m.
Reward/Consequence	Success for the week earns a movie night on Friday. If this goal is not met, there is no screen time at all for the weekend.

Monday	Tuesday	Wednesday	Thursday	Friday	Goal Met
Yes	X	Yes	X	Yes	Yes

Homework blueprint:

Goal	Complete eight minutes of homework daily between 4:00 and 7:00 p.m. One pass card issued for a "free pass" night. Amanda can choose the night she'd like to skip.
Reward/Consequence	Success for the week earns one downloadable song. No screen time until the homework goal is met each night. No screen time for the day if the daily homework goal is not met.

Monday	Tuesday	Wednesday	Thursday	Friday	Goal Met
Pass Card	Yes	Yes	Yes	Yes	Yes

The following week Amanda made small gains toward both of her goals: she increased her time at school, staying until 1:00 p.m. three days per week, and she began doing eleven minutes a night of homework. She continued to have one pass for the nurse each day and one pass for homework for the week. Her stepwise progress in all of these

Amanda's second week.

School attendance blueprint:

Goal:	Go to school Monday, Wednesday, and Friday until 1:00 p.m.
Reward/Consequence	Success for the week earns a movie night on Friday. If this goal is not met, there is no screen time at all for the weekend.

Monday	Tuesday	Wednesday	Thursday	Friday	Goal Met
Yes	X	Yes	X	Yes (Stayed all day at school)	Yes

Homework blueprint:

Goal	Complete 11 minutes of homework between 4:00 and 7:00 p.m.
Reward/Consequence	80% success for the week earns one downloadable song. No screen time until homework goal is met each night. No screen time for the day if daily homework goal not met.

Monday	Tuesday	Wednesday	Thursday	Friday	Goal Met
Yes	Pass Card	X	Yes	Yes	No

areas meant that she was feeling increasingly confident that she could be successful overall.

Amanda actually exceeded her attendance goal by staying all day on the Friday of the second week. While she wasn't pressured to stay longer, there was a school assembly that she wanted to attend, so she

Amanda's third week.

School attendance blueprint:

Goal	Go to school Monday, Tuesday, Thursday and Friday until 1:00 p.m.
Reward/Consequence	Success for the week earns a movie night on Friday. If this goal is not met, there is no screen time at all for the weekend.

Monday	Tuesday	Wednesday	Thursday	Friday	Goal Met
Yes	Yes	No	Yes	Yes	Yes

Homework blueprint:

Goal	Complete 15 minutes of homework between 4:00 and 7:00 p.m.
Reward/Consequence	80% success for the week earns one download-able song. No screen time until homework goal is met each night. No screen time for the day if the daily homework goal is not met.

Monday	Tuesday	Wednesday	Thursday	Friday	Goal Met
Yes	Yes	Yes	Yes	Pass card	Yes

was encouraged to do so. Amanda did not do as well on her homework goals. Amanda used her pass card on Tuesday night, but failed her goal on Wednesday night. Even though Amanda said that she was tired from being at school on Wednesday and had increased pain, her parents held her accountable and she lost screen time for twenty-four hours. At the end of the week, she earned her reward for attendance (movie night), but *not* the one for homework (a downloadable song).

Amanda's fourth week.

School attendance blueprint:

Goal	Go to school every day until 1:00 p.m.
Reward/Consequence	Success for the week earns a movie night on Friday. If this goal is not met, there is no screen time at all for the weekend.

Monday	Tuesday	Wednesday	Thursday	Friday	Goal Met
Yes	X	X	X	X	No

Homework blueprint:

Goal	Complete 20 minutes of homework between 4:00 and 7:00 p.m.
Reward/Consequence	80% success for the week earns one download-able song. No screen time until homework goal is met each night. No screen time for the day if the daily homework goal is not met.

Monday	Tuesday	Wednesday	Thursday	Friday	Goal Met
Pass Card	Yes	Yes	Yes	Yes	Yes

The following week the attendance goals were set for Amanda to attend four days per week and stay until 1:00 p.m. Her homework-time goal increased to fifteen minutes a day.

Amanda had great success in her third week. At this point, three weeks into her school plan, she had developed some confidence that she could continue to slowly increase her time at school. Moreover, she was motivated to complete her fifteen minutes of homework a night in order to maintain screen time and gain her reward. Her parents shared the happy news with the school and celebrated Amanda's successful week at home.

By week four the plan was for Amanda to attend five days a week until 1:00 p.m. Her homework was increased to twenty minutes per night, and she maintained her pass cards for school and home.

Week four was not a good week, but setbacks like these are not at all uncommon. Right when things are starting to go well and get back on track, the plan feels like it falls apart. Sometimes, plans fall flat when a child gets sick with the flu, has medical appointments in the middle of the day, experiences a really tough pain flare, or just loses motivation. Whatever the reason, it's important not to get discouraged.

In Amanda's case, she had a pain flare. Because her attendance goal was not met, she lost all screen time for the weekend including her movie night. But she did maintain an hour of screen time per evening during the week for completing her homework goal and earned her downloadable song. While talking about the missed attendance goal, Amanda was able to make a link between feeling stressed about increasing demands at school and the onset of her pain. Amanda was encouraged to think about using additional relaxation skills and increasing her moderate exercise to help manage this stress.

Despite the setback in Amanda's attendance, the plan moved forward. At this point, however, Amanda asked that instead of increasing the frequency of her days at school, she be allowed to increase the length of time she was at school and preserve one day off in her week. Her parents agreed, changing her blueprint so that she was scheduled to attend four days a week until 2:00 p.m. She was also given an additional pass card (two in all) for taking breaks with the nurse as needed during her longer day. Feeling that Amanda could increase the frequency of her homework time, her parents let her know that if she didn't use her homework pass card she could cash it in at the end of the week for a special dinner reward; Amanda chose the incentive of earning pancakes for dinner.

Amanda's fifth and final week.

School attendance blueprint:

Goal:	Go to school Monday, Tuesday, Thursday, and Friday until 2:00 p.m.
Reward/Consequence	Success for the week earns a movie night on Friday. If this goal is not met, there is no screen time at all for the weekend.

Monday	Tuesday	Wednesday	Thursday	Friday	Goal Met
Yes	Yes	X	Yes	Yes	Yes

Homework blueprint:

Goal	Complete 25 minutes of homework between 4:00 and 7:00 p.m.
Reward/Consequence	80% success for the week earns one downloadable song. No screen time until the homework goal is met each night. No screen time for the day if the daily homework goal is not met. Bonus: can cash in pass card for a pancake dinner.

Monday	Tuesday	Wednesday	Thursday	Friday	Goal Met
Yes	Yes	Yes	Yes	Yes	Yes

The fifth week of the blueprint was Amanda's best week in school since September. She earned her rewards for attendance and homework, earned pancakes for dinner for not using her homework pass card, and felt proud of her progress. Though it took five weeks to get to this point, and setbacks had occurred, with the structure of the school plan, the confidence that comes from having prepared carefully for the return to school, parent collaboration and support, accommodations at school, and good problem-solving skills, Amanda was clearly getting back on track. She continued to make slow but steady progress until she was attending five full school days a week and doing all of her homework for a minimum of one hour every night.

◆

How to Help

1. DEVELOP A GOOD RELATIONSHIP WITH SCHOOL STAFF

Parents should approach all school interactions with an understanding that the school staff may have limited knowledge about chronic pain conditions. Parents should also be willing to compromise and try various solutions, and to work hard to keep communications wide open. Remember that parents' goodwill toward the school and the school staff not only will make working together easier and probably more productive, but also will help their child have a positive attitude toward school.

2. BE PREPARED TO EDUCATE THE SCHOOL STAFF

Parents should assume that the school staff have had little opportunity to work with a child who has chronic pain. As a starting point, parents should obtain documentation from doctors and from trusted websites that will lay the groundwork for those teachers and other school professionals who may be unfamiliar with a child's diagnosis or pain difficulty.

3. WORK WITH THE SCHOOL NURSE

The school nurse can be a valuable ally and support for your child while your child is at school. The key is to meet with the nurse as early as possible to ensure that he or she fully understands your child's pain problem and knows how to support your child during the school day. You might suggest a system of fifteen-minute breaks or the "pass-card" system discussed in this chapter. Then be sure your child and the school nurse also have a chance to develop their own strong partnership, to help ensure that your child will always have a friendly, knowledgeable person to turn to during the school day.

4. REQUEST A FORMAL SCHOOL PLAN IF NEEDED

If a school is not being responsive to requests for accommodation or support, parents should not be shy about requesting a formal school plan. In most states, these requests must be in writing and schools have a mandate to respond to this request within a specified time frame.

5. DEVELOP A BLUEPRINT FOR SCHOOL-RELATED GOALS

Work with your child to identify one or two goals related to attending school or completing schoolwork. Set clear guidelines for success and make sure that everyone knows what will happen if she or he does not follow the plan. Plan to work toward these school goals in small increments and be on the lookout for school-specific factors (learning issues, peer issues, environmental issues) that may be barriers to progress.

6. DEVISE AN IN-SCHOOL COPING PLAN WITH YOUR CHILD

All the relaxation skills you helped your child to develop can be a very important part of an in-school coping plan. Kids can often use diaphragmatic breathing or mindfulness to relax and reduce symptoms in the classroom without peers or teachers even noticing. A plan to engage in a pre-recorded (or apps-based) guided-imagery or progressive-muscle-relaxation exercise during a nurse visit can maximize the benefit of taking this break from the classroom environment (see Appendix 3 for suggestions of apps to try). Other coping skills such as finding a friend to talk to for distraction or taking a walking or stretching break can also be helpful. Make sure your child can identify a clear plan for how he or she intends to cope with discomfort while at school.

7. ONCE A SCHOOL PLAN IS IN PLACE, STEP BACK

The beauty of a clear school blueprint is that parents don't have to nag, persuade, or beg their child to cooperate. Part of the plan should be for kids to take responsibility for getting up in the morning and preparing to go to school. Additionally, while a single gentle reminder to do homework may be helpful, parents should not have to continually remind their child to do homework. When parents step back, kids will have the choice to either step up and meet their goal, or deal with the planned consequence of not meeting that goal. This is often a monumental shift for families, and importantly, one that can set the stage for kids taking a more active role in their recovery, thus fueling greater success.

8. ADDITIONAL READING

For more on helping your child do his or her best in school, take a look at the 2007 book by Christopher Kearney, a specialist in this area, entitled *Getting Your Child to Say "Yes" to School.*

17

Reversing the Habits of Poor Sleep

From the time our children are born, we are preoccupied with their sleep. As parents, we all learn that a lack of sleep can have disastrous effects. No parent wants to deal with a cranky or irritable child, so we work fervently to make sure our children get to sleep at a reasonable time each night and have enough rest to make it through their busy days. You've probably noticed, too, how your child's sleeping habits have changed. Sleep patterns change rapidly over the first year of life. Then, as a toddler, your child probably settled into a pattern of sleeping about ten hours a night and taking one to two naps per day. Between the ages of five and twelve, children usually get the best nighttime sleep they will have in their whole life. Melatonin, a hormone we release during our nighttime sleep cycle, is at an all-time high during these ages so children can often fall asleep quickly and sleep ten to fourteen hours a night. In contrast, while adolescents still typically require nine to ten hours of sleep per night, they are challenged with hormonal changes that routinely alter their circadian rhythms. Most adolescents find that they can no longer fall asleep early and, often to their parents' frustration, prefer to sleep late into the morning (or afternoon). In a population of healthy adolescents, only 50 percent report that they had a good night's sleep and feel well rested. Moreover, approximately one in four adolescents reports that they are chronically sleep deprived, attaining fewer than six hours of sleep per night.

It is worrisome to read the latest research on the discrepancy between the amount of sleep that children and adolescents need for optimal growth and development and the amount of sleep they are actually attaining. Because sleep deprivation in late childhood and adolescence is such a common phenomenon, one might think that it's a normal part of development. But this just isn't the case. Kids who do not consistently attain adequate sleep have been documented to be at greater risk for obesity, diabetes, depression, and even suicide. Moreover, poor sleep causes a global reduction in academic performance with noted impairments in memory, concentration, and problem-solving skills. Lack of sleep is also related to decreased immune functioning, meaning that sleep-deprived children are more likely to get sick than their well-rested peers. Over the past ten years, studies have also found that a lack of sleep may be a primary cause of inflammation and pain. Research shows that cytokines, a type of protein released by cells that can trigger pain, are more prevalent in people who are sleep-deprived. Along these same lines of research, there is evidence suggesting that chronic sleep difficulties may be a significant risk factor in the development of autoimmune diseases. This compelling body of research underscores the importance of addressing sleep deficits, especially for children who have pain.

More than 40 percent of children who have chronic pain report struggling with sleep disturbances as well. This is a huge obstacle for parents and children. Poor sleep is stressful for kids and parents alike, and research has shown that children with pain who do not sleep well have more significant difficulties getting back to school and activities and experience an overall poorer quality of life. Pain symptoms often make it difficult for children to get comfortable and fall asleep at night, so it's not surprising that poor sleep and resulting daytime fatigue are among the most common complaints associated with pain. But the relationship between sleep and pain is far more complex than this. A lack of sleep contributes to increased sensitivity to pain, and pain is associated with general hyperarousal and hypervigilance, physiological states that lead to the release of hormones that can also interfere with falling sleep and staying asleep.

Children with pain very quickly fall into poor sleep patterns, and over time, these poor patterns become habits. Once disrupted sleep becomes a habit for the body, it is difficult to restore good sleep. But good sleep is vitally important: it can reduce pain in children and help them return to normal daily activities even when pain persists, in part because rested children feel more prepared emotionally and physically to tackle the challenges of the day.

There are several kinds of sleep disruptions, including difficulty falling asleep, difficulty staying asleep, and daytime fatigue. In this chapter we will first review some general guidelines for securing a good night's rest, and then detail how to address specific problem areas related to sleep habits.

Sleep Cycles

A basic understanding of sleep cycles is enormously helpful when working to modify and address issues of poor sleep. While there are developmental differences in terms of exactly how long particular sleep cycles last, the general framework of sleep, or one's "sleep architecture," is fairly consistent throughout a person's life. A person's sleep architecture can be displayed in a graph called a hypnogram, which shows how much time a person spends in each sleep stage and how the stages change over the course of a typical night. In addition to the rapid eye movement (REM) stage, there are four sleep stages, which range from stage 1, the shallowest sleep stage, to stage 4, the deepest sleep. Restorative rest takes place during stages 3 and 4.

Understanding this architecture will illuminate how best to help children improve their sleep habits. Along the left side of the sample hypnogram you can see the stages of sleep and on the bottom you can see the number of hours of sleep. In the course of a typical eight-hour night

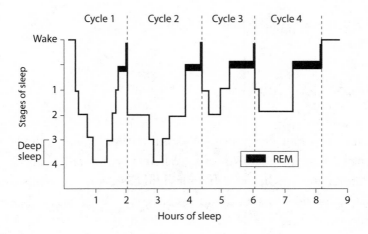

A graph of an entire sleep cycle, also known as a hypnogram.

of sleep, a person will experience three to four full sleep cycles. Following along from the left to the right you can see that within one hour of falling asleep, a child passes from wakefulness to stage 4 sleep, and by about the one-and-a-half hour mark, the child has cycled back up to REM sleep. During REM sleep our brains are very active and close to waking, so it is common for people to wake up briefly during a stage of REM sleep, which occurs three to four times per night. The second half of the night, from about the three-hour mark until the eight-hour mark, is characterized by longer episodes of deep sleep. Deep sleep is very restorative and most people do not arouse easily from it. Importantly, the amount of time a child spends in this part of sleep can vary based on need. So if a child has a restless night of sleep on a Thursday, on Friday night he or she will probably spend more time in deep sleep to make up for the deficit, even if the overall hours of sleep don't change. This is important because it means that children don't have to make up every lost hour of sleep. The body knows to compensate for a wakeful night with more deep sleep later, and to some extent this helps to mitigate the loss of sleep and the fatigue that results from having too little sleep.

The amount of sleep needed to feel well rested varies among individuals. But for almost everyone experiencing chronic pain, significant disruptions to sleep can throw off a steady recovery. Fortunately, there are many proven strategies for improving sleep that can easily be tried at home.

General Sleep Guidelines

Just as good dental hygiene involves routine healthy behaviors like brushing, flossing, and rinsing, healthy sleep requires good "sleep hygiene"—healthy habits designed to help a person fall asleep and stay asleep for a good night's rest. If your child has disrupted sleep, the first thing you can do is ensure that these sleep hygiene goals are being met as fully as possible.

1. *No napping.* While poor nighttime sleep often results in fatigue during the day, naps tend to do more harm than good. Within an hour of falling asleep the body slips into stage 4 deep sleep (see the earlier hypnogram), so waking up after a one-hour nap can be extremely difficult, and instead of feeling refreshed from the nap, most people feel groggy for several hours. Even worse, napping an hour or more can trick the body into thinking that it already had good sleep, which means that falling asleep in the evening is much harder to do. My stalwart advice is no napping during the day if a child is not sleeping well at night. If your child *absolutely* must take a nap, he or she should be limited to no more than a thirty-minute "power nap." This short nap does not generally allow the body to shift into deeper stages of sleep, so he or she can reawaken more easily from the nap and is more likely to feel refreshed.
2. *End all screen time at least one hour before bed.* Not only are computers, smartphones, video games, and TVs very stimulating for the brain; the light they give off interferes with the release of the hormone melatonin. Melatonin is a naturally occurring hormone that is released when it gets dark outside, to signal to the brain that it's time for sleep. When the eyes are exposed to bright light, especially the blue light that is emitted from screens, the release of melatonin is delayed, making it more difficult to go to sleep.

3. *Plan a set wake-up time every morning.* Even if a child's nighttime sleep is disrupted, it's important to wake up at the same time each morning. Sleeping late often seems like the antidote to staying up late, but when kids get in the habit of sleeping late they can inadvertently shift their whole sleep cycle, making it increasingly more difficult to fall asleep at night (see the information on delayed sleep phase disorder later in this chapter).

4. *Don't lie awake in bed all night.* If your child can't sleep, suggest that he or she get out of bed and for the next twenty minutes either read with a small book light or do another quiet, non-screen-related activity, then try to go to sleep again. Staying in bed for hours and not sleeping can be stressful and can lead children to associate their bed with not sleeping.

5. *Use the bed only for sleep.* Many adolescents get in the habit of using their bed to do homework, watch TV, or other activities. If your child is not sleeping well, it's important that he or she retrain their brain to think of bed only as a place for sleep. If needed, work with your child to create another cozy spot in the house for doing all of the other activities and make the bed a peaceful and sacred place reserved for sleep.

6. *Set an optimal sleeping environment.* To the extent possible make your child's bedroom environment conducive to sleep. Make sure the light is blocked from the windows and hall, consider using a white noise machine or have your child use soft foam earplugs if there is a lot of noise in the house at bedtime, keep the room cool, and make sure your child has comfortable pillows and blankets.

7. *Avoid caffeine.* There should be a strict rule of no caffeine after lunchtime. Even if your adolescent says "caffeine doesn't affect me," late afternoon or evening caffeine can impair the brain's ability to ease into sleep.

8. *Remove clocks, phones, and all screens.* Yes, kids will fight you on this. But if your child is not sleeping well, you should steadfastly keep technology out of his or her bedroom. Removing clocks helps to reduce the stress of seeing how late it is, and removing phones

and screens eliminates the temptation to engage in screen time or connect with peers. Research shows that the mere presence of a TV in a child's room (not necessarily the quantity of TV watched) is associated with thirty minutes less sleep per night when compared to children who do not have TVs in their room.

9. *Exercise.* Daytime exercise is linked to better nighttime sleep. Ideally daily exercise should include at least twenty minutes of aerobic activity, but even a short walk or bike ride can help. If your child is physically not able to walk around, he or she may be able to do upper-body exercises or a series of yoga stretches to get the heart pumping. One caveat: be sure not to exercise within two hours of bedtime. The body needs adequate time to cool down before it can drift into sleep.

Difficulty Falling Asleep

Many children with pain have difficulty falling asleep. Whether this problem is due to the pain itself, pain-related stressors, or the habit of poor sleep matters very little in terms of how we work to alleviate this difficulty. If your child is having difficulty falling asleep at night, it will be worthwhile to try some intervention strategies that can help to reduce pain, ease stress, and undo the habit of getting into bed and *not* sleeping.

First, establish a bedtime routine that starts about one hour before your child will actually get into bed. This means that kids will need to stop homework and screen time, and start preparing for bed, one hour before he or she would like to fall asleep. A bedtime routine may include soothing strategies such as a warm bath or shower, a light non-sugary snack, some chamomile tea, the use of soothing aromatherapy scents such as lavender, and some quiet time to read. During this time you can even dim the lights to prepare the brain and body for sleep. It's important to keep in mind that if your child is routinely not falling asleep until 1:00 a.m., starting a bedtime routine at 8:00 p.m. is not likely to be successful. Think about when your child is actually falling asleep and aim for a bedtime that is just slightly earlier, then work incrementally from there. For example, for a child who is not falling asleep until 1:00 a.m., I would suggest that a one-hour bedtime routine not start until 11:00 p.m. This way by 11:45 p.m. or midnight your child will be ready to get into bed and is more likely to fall asleep quickly. Once your child has adjusted to the new routine and is successful with the earlier bedtime, you can continue to shift bedtime earlier by twenty to thirty minutes every week until you feel like a healthy bedtime is in place.

If worries are a problem for your child, have your child keep a pen and paper by his or her bed. Encourage your child to do a "brain dump" before bed, writing down as many of the concerns or problems that come to mind. This brief exercise can help to calm your child's mind while he or she is trying to fall asleep.

After a bedtime routine and a "brain dump" comes relaxation. Bedtime is the perfect time to engage in any of the relaxation strategies detailed in Part 3. Initially, it can be helpful for parents to lead these exercises with their child, but if or when your child prefers to practice these exercises independently, that is also fine. Even when parents start off leading the exercises, if children are older than age eight, parents should eventually ease themselves out of the bedtime relaxation routine. When parents step back it empowers kids to learn to prepare for bed on their own, boosting confidence in their ability to manage pain and stress. Even more importantly, if parents are needed as part of a prolonged soothing process every night to help a child fall asleep, when a child wakes up in the middle of the night he or she will likely need a parent again to get back to sleep. In contrast, a child who has learned to self-soothe at the start of the night is more likely to be able to self-soothe in the middle of the night and fall back to sleep without parent assistance.

Parents and kids should commit to following these bedtime guidelines for at least fourteen consecutive days before determining if they are working. I always encourage children and parents to record their progress on a chart so that they can track what time a child went to bed and how quickly he or she fell asleep. Keep in mind that as with other behavioral changes, progress is measured in small steps and isn't always linear. In other words, it's not uncommon to have a good night getting to sleep followed by a bad night. It takes a while to undo the pattern of having difficulty falling asleep, so be patient.

Waking Up at Night

Nighttime waking is common for children who have pain, in part because stress hormones that accompany pain and pain-related stress can be released at night and these can interrupt sleep cycles. Additionally, if children are physically uncomfortable, when they cycle through to phases of light sleep (stage 1 and REM, which occur three to four times per night), they may wake up from their discomfort. For these reasons, its very common for kids to report that they wake up at least once, but often as many as four or more times, per night. Parents and kids begin to understand the cycle of repeated waking when I show them the hypnogram and explain the physiology of sleep; what to do about it is sometimes less clear.

The first thing I like to let kids know is that if they are occasionally waking up briefly and falling back to sleep without much difficulty, they shouldn't worry about the fact that they are waking up. It's common for people to awaken briefly during their light sleep-cycle phases. In fact, as we grow older, it becomes increasingly more common to have these brief awakenings. Fortunately, these brief periods of alertness in the middle of the night don't appear to significantly impair the overall quality of sleep. So if kids wake during their light sleep cycles and fall back to sleep within ten to fifteen minutes, don't worry. These disruptions can be related to pain, stress, growth spurts, or other triggers and will likely not significantly interfere with their progress in other areas of their recovery.

If nighttime awakenings are frequent or lead to longer periods of alertness, there are a few key "sleep hygiene" tactics to keep in mind. Remember not to turn on bright lights, including any screens, in the middle of the night, which could trick the brain into thinking that it's morning and so could suppress the release of melatonin and make it much more difficult to fall back asleep. Also children should avoid drinking too much water or other fluids at least one hour before bedtime because the urge to urinate can wake a child.

Beyond maintaining good sleep hygiene, it's also important to have a plan to deal with nighttime waking. For example, if kids wake up in the night they should first be encouraged to remain in bed and try some of the diaphragmatic breathing strategies described in Chapter 10. Breathing in and out one time for each letter in a child's name or taking one deep breath for each year the child is old can often be enough to soothe a child back into sleep. If that doesn't work, the middle of the night is a good time to listen to an audio-based relaxation strategy such as a guided-imagery story (see Chapter 11) or passive progressive-muscle-relaxation exercise (see Chapter 12). If a child still can't sleep, he or she should get out of bed and try a quiet activity in another part of the house. For example, a child can turn on a small book light and read for twenty minutes. At the end of the twenty minutes, the child can return to bed, try a relaxation strategy, and then attempt to fall asleep again. Having a plan that a child can carry out on her own can reduce the need for parents to be awakened for all episodes of nighttime sleeplessness.

It's ideal for kids to quietly and independently manage their nighttime wakefulness. But this is a learned skill and, at least initially, this won't come easily for many children. So what should parents do when their child frequently wakes them up in the middle of the night?

Parent Involvement

There are many ways that parents get woven into the fabric of their child's sleep disruption. Some children and even older adolescents simply crawl into bed with their parents in the middle of the night and spend their night there. Some parents crawl into bed with their kids. Other kids don't want to sleep with their parents, but do want their parents' attention in the middle of the night. Some parents are just light sleepers and wake up when their child wakes up at night, then get caught up worrying about or caring for their child and can't fall back asleep.

There are many ways to approach these challenges. But the very first thing parents need to keep in mind is that when they are sleep deprived, they are much less effective when helping their child during the day. Sleep deprivation can lead to health problems in adults such as diabetes, heart disease, and obesity. Moreover, far more car accidents occur when adults are sleep deprived and the ability to solve problems decreases dramatically. For these reasons, this is one of the situations when parents need to follow the instructions given on every major airline: take care of yourself first—put that oxygen mask on—and then assist your child. Most kids can safely and effectively make it through the night without your active involvement and you will be a better, calmer, more effective parent if you prioritize your own sleep. An exception to this is if your child requires medication dosing at night. In this case, parents may need to wake up and administer the medication so that mistakes aren't made.

CO-SLEEPING

I fully support co-sleeping by parents and their young children if this is part of the family culture. If co-sleeping works in your family—meaning that kids and parents both obtain quality, restful sleep, they both enjoy the experience, and you would co-sleep even if your child's pain or medical stress weren't an issue—then certainly this can be maintained. But it doesn't work for every kid or parent, and it certainly becomes more challenging as kids get bigger. When Dad has been relegated to the couch to make room for Mom to sleep with a teenage daughter in the master bed, or when Mom's neck and shoulders are perpetually sore from being crammed in the corner of her son's twin bed, or whenever a child or parent is not sleeping soundly, then co-sleeping is not working.

Many older kids and adolescents don't necessarily want to sleep with their parents; they just want a parent to witness the difficulty they are having. It can feel very lonely to be up in the middle of the night and unable to go back to sleep, and when pain is the cause, kids often crave a parent's soothing touch or simply a parent's presence. While parents recognize this, they feel helpless to do much in the middle of the night and increasingly feel frustrated with the routine nighttime awakenings. If parents would like to reduce or eliminate the experience of having their child wake them in the middle of the night, they should forge ahead and leave feelings of guilt behind. Older kids and adolescents can certainly learn to manage their own nighttime wakefulness and you will feel much better yourself if you can obtain a better rest.

SETTING A NEW COURSE

To undo the habits of parent involvement at night, the first thing you have to do is let your child know that this situation is not working and that you need to make changes to ensure that you get your rest and can continue to help him during the day. Next pick a stretch of a week or two when you can commit to, in the worst-case scenario, being totally sleep deprived. Of course, there is no time that will seem like a good time to do this, and it will often seem far easier just to let this pattern continue. But dedicating a few days to this cause can lead to much better sleep on the other end; a pretty good incentive. Once you've set the stage for an intervention and picked a time to start it, the next thing is to do is make the blueprint.

A Blueprint to Reduce Parent Involvement at Night

Many parents may recall the wisdom of Richard Ferber, who made behavioral conditioning a staple approach to consolidating infant sleep. Ferber's approach has sometimes had the unfortunate misnomer of the "cry-it-out" method. In fact, when done correctly at the right age and stage of development, there is very little crying involved. Moreover, with this method within one to two weeks crying at night is almost eliminated and infants emerge as happy, healthy sleepers. While kids with pain and infants have very different needs, the same behavioral conditioning approach can be used to reduce the amount of time that parents spend with their child at bedtime and eliminate the routine occurrence of kids waking their parents in the middle of the night.

Like any functional behavior change, it's best to "scaffold" the approach—work it out in a systematic, detailed way so you and your child can feel confident that it will be successful. Sit down with your child and figure out on average how many times he or she wakes you in the middle of the night. Then think through how your parent involvement can be slowly and steadily lessened over time. Be sure to brainstorm with your child ideas for nighttime self-care, and create together a personal plan for coping with pain or stress at bedtime or in the middle of the night. Remember that it may take several weeks to establish new habits that don't include parental help—be patient and understanding, even as you stick to your plan for at least fourteen days.

The Case of Peter

Peter, a fifteen-year-old boy, was diagnosed with juvenile arthritis and pain amplification syndrome nine months before first seeing me. Since his symptoms appeared, his sleep had been very disrupted. He was waking up in the middle of the night at least once, and frequently two or three times. Once he was awake he became anxious about his lack of sleep and worried about how tired he would be the next day. This made it increasingly difficult for him to go back to sleep. Peter had fallen into the habit of waking his Mom each time he woke up. Initially she didn't mind being awakened and in fact encouraged him to seek her support. But her mounting exhaustion and the fact that there was little she could offer her teenage son in the middle of the night led to their decision to change this habit.

Tracking how many times per night Peter woke his Mom revealed that he was waking her on average at least two times a night (fourteen times a week) and that they were co-sleeping in her bed approximately one night per week. Using a scaffolded stepwise approach, they decided to start their plan by scaling back the number of times he was waking her per week by four. So in the first week, he was allowed to wake his Mom only ten times (instead of fourteen). Given that Peter was fifteen years old, he was okay with eliminating altogether the one night of co-sleeping.

Before starting this sleep plan, Peter and his Mom developed a series of coping strategies for his nighttime pain and awakening. Peter agreed to first try deep-breathing exercises to relax and to use a heating pad (kept next to his bed) on his joints if he had discomfort. He also kept his iTouch and a set of headphones just outside his bedroom door so that he could access a guided-imagery app to further relax his mind and ease discomfort if needed. If that didn't work, he would try gently massaging his joints and reading quietly on the family room couch with a book light. After reading three chapters he would return to his bed and try to sleep again. He was encouraged to write down notes about how long he was awake if he wanted to share that information with his Mom the next day.

Peter was then given a stack of ten nighttime passes. Each time he woke his Mom, he cashed in a pass. He had to budget the use of these throughout the week. If he woke his Mom *after* using up all of his passes (that is, if he failed to stick to the plan), he would lose the privilege of having his Mom make his lunch for school the next day. This meant that Peter would either have to wake up earlier in the morning (allowing his mother to sleep longer) to prepare his own lunch or eat the school lunch, which he disliked. As an incentive to work hard with this plan, he and his Mom agreed that he could keep his unused nighttime passes at the end of each week. When he collected fifteen unused passes, he could earn tickets to go hear his favorite band perform.

During the first week Peter was very successful, using only seven of his ten night passes. He reserved the three leftover passes to put toward his concert tickets. The next week Peter was given only eight passes for the week. He used only four and had four passes to put toward

Peter's sleep blueprint.

Goal	Wake mom at night no more than 10 times in one week
Reward/Consequence	Unused passes count as points toward concert tickets. (15 unused passes = one concert ticket). Waking mom after using all 10 passes means you have to make your own lunch in the morning (or eat school lunch).

Monday	Tuesday	Wednesday	Thursday	Friday	Saturday	Sunday	Total
2	0	1	1	0	2	1	7 passes used

his tickets. The following week he was issued only six passes, and he used five. The week after that he was given five passes and used only two. The week after that he was given four passes and didn't use any of them.

Peter's Mom reported that she felt much better with this plan in place. While she was initially still being awakened many times per week via the pass card system, knowing that there was a plan and seeing the progress early on helped her to feel that there was a light at the end of the tunnel. Even more important, she was sleeping more, which reduced her overall fatigue and irritability. Peter also reported that he was benefiting from the plan. After five weeks, Peter was still waking frequently, but falling back to sleep much more quickly than when he was waking his Mom at night. Practicing his self-soothing techniques and involving his Mom less increased his confidence that he could manage his nighttime waking. Six weeks into the plan Peter earned his concert tickets. The following week Peter gained the confidence to stay overnight at his best friend's house, something he had been unable to do for more than a year.

Medical Conditions That Disrupt Sleep

While pain, pain-related stress, and poor sleep habits can all lead to restless and ineffectual sleep at night, it is also true that poor sleep can cause many health problems, including sore muscles and joints, headaches, memory and concentration issues, chronic fatigue, dizziness, anxiety, depression, and weight gain. If your child was a poor sleeper prior to the onset of pain, or if your child experiences any of the signs or symptoms described here, you should discuss these issues with your child's doctor. Treatment recommendations specific to sleep disorders, or a visit to a pediatric sleep center, may be warranted.

OBSTRUCTIVE SLEEP APNEA

Sleep apnea occurs when a person's airway becomes constricted while sleeping at night. For people who have this disorder, this airway constriction can lead to hundreds of nighttime arousals. These mini-awakenings may or may not cause a person to wake up fully, but they definitely interfere with the attainment of deep sleep and thus lead to chronic sleep deprivation. Sleep apnea is commonly thought of as a problem that only occurs in middle-aged, overweight men, but 5 percent of children and adolescents also struggle with this condition. The primary red flag for sleep apnea is snoring so loud that it can often be heard in another room. Sleep apnea can produce a pattern of snoring interrupted by brief periods of silence, then followed by gasps or snorting sounds. If your child has this pattern of breathing, bring these concerns to the attention of your child's doctor. If your child is overweight, he or she may be at increased risk.

BRUXISM

Bruxism is the medical term for grinding teeth. The primary red flag for bruxism is the sound of very loud grinding while a person sleeps at night; the noise is similar to the sound of rocks rubbing together. Bruxism can be an underlying cause for headaches, temporomandibular joint dysfunction (TMJ), ear or face pain, and dental-related problems such as cracks in teeth or fillings. Bruxism in children may resolve without treatment, but if you notice that your child grinds his or her teeth at night, you should notify your child's doctor.

DELAYED SLEEP PHASE DISORDER

This disorder characterizes the night owl: a person who "comes alive" at night, doesn't feel sleepy until around 3:00 a.m., and is then very difficult to awaken in the morning. While this may seem to describe every teenager, a true phase disorder can cause a significant amount of distress and disruption in daily activities. People with this disorder may be extremely fatigued and groggy well into midday and they often don't respond well to typical sleep hygiene strategies. Modifying a phase disorder can often be accomplished with a structured behavioral plan that includes stringent sleep-wake times, exposure to either natural light or a light box early in the morning, daily exercise, and the use of melatonin at night (see the next paragraphs). Working closely with a primary care or behavioral health provider can be very useful for modifying this type of sleep disorder.

THE POTENTIAL BENEFITS OF MELATONIN

If your child persistently struggles to fall asleep and hasn't responded to a solid trial of behavioral recommendations, you may want to consider a trial with synthetic melatonin. Melatonin is a hormone that naturally occurs in our body and is released at night when our eyes are exposed to dark. Supplementing with synthetic melatonin is thought to help induce sleep.

When melatonin first became widely available in the 1990s it was praised as a highly effective sleep aid for everyone. Research has failed to fully back up this claim. Melatonin does seem to work for a subset of people, especially those who have a delayed sleep phase disorder. Though melatonin is available over the counter in the United States, if you would like to initiate a trial of melatonin, you should first consult your child's doctor.

Parents should keep in mind that melatonin is generally recommended only for short-term use; the effects of taking melatonin for months or years are not well known. As a general rule, children should start a trial of melatonin with the lowest dose possible to obtain the desired effect. It's recommended that kids take the supplement approximately thirty minutes before bedtime, but always before 10:00 p.m. because a later dose may make it difficult to wake up in the morning. There are infrequent side effects associated with melatonin, but dizziness, nausea, and headache have been reported in some research studies.

◆

How to Help

1. TEACH YOUR CHILD THE BASICS ABOUT SLEEP HEALTH

Share information with your child about normal sleep patterns and the ways in which pain can interfere. Talk with your child about what part of the night is the hardest for him or her and target that area first.

2. THINK OF POOR SLEEP AS A HABIT OF THE BODY

While pain, hormones, medications, or stress may all have been initial factors in a disrupted sleep pattern, quite frequently the persistence of poor sleep is, at least in part, a bad habit for the body. Reversing this habit takes time; in fact, it can take two or more weeks to form new, healthier sleep habits.

3. GET SERIOUS ABOUT SLEEP HYGIENE

Most teenagers roll their eyes when I review sleep hygiene. Many have heard some or all of the sleep hygiene advice before and quickly dismiss it before they give it a try. But when I really hold kids accountable for making these changes, the feedback I get (albeit begrudgingly) is that they work. Beyond my clinical experience, research confirms that when kids do actually make recommended changes to their sleep hygiene, lasting improvements are evident.

4. WORK WITH YOUR CHILD TO DEVELOP A NIGHTTIME COPING PLAN

Talking about a coping plan for the middle of the night, or even better, writing it down, can help to eliminate unhelpful behaviors such as ruminating at night about not sleeping, waking parents for support, or trying to come up with a plan while exhausted during the night. Nighttime plans should ideally include a one-hour pre-bedtime routine to help relax into sleep, a plan for managing restlessness once in bed, and a plan for nighttime awakenings. Nighttime plans should include quiet, soothing, non-screen-based approaches for relaxation.

5. RECLAIM PARENT SLEEP

Remember that parents who sleep better are healthier and have a greater capacity to help their child during the day. If that's not enough reason to decrease parent involvement at night, consider that parent attention at nighttime can unintentionally reinforce a child's sleep disruptions. So talk with your kids about decreasing your involvement at night. Set up a blueprint to wean your child from the habit of waking a parent at night and consider rewarding your child for success with this goal.

6. TALK WITH YOUR CHILD'S DOCTOR ABOUT A PLAN FOR SLEEP

Most physicians routinely inquire about a child's sleep because having restful, regular sleep is such an integral part of a child's health and well-being. First-line treatments for any problems usually include the behavioral sleep-hygiene strategies suggested in this chapter. Persistent sleep disruptions that do not respond to behavioral modifications, however, may warrant a trial of melatonin, changes to a medication plan, or possibly a referral for a sleep study.

18

Where Are My Child's Friends?

If you are a parent of a child with chronic pain, I probably don't have to tell you that having chronic pain can be a lonely and alienating experience for a child. Between 40 and 60 percent of children with pain report that they are having some problems with their social relationships or have stopped doing activities that keep them in touch with friends. As a parent, you probably recognize that fitting in with peers is a very important goal for your child. Indeed, research shows that support and validation from friendships are essential for developing self-esteem and a positive sense of self-worth.

Unfortunately, many children with pain and medical stress are less active with friends and may lose important social connections. This happens in part because children with chronic pain are frequently absent from school and often have limited participation in sports or other extracurricular activities. Children with chronic pain or illness may also choose to withdraw from friends or activities if they feel that their symptoms make them look physically different or in some other way make them stand out from others. Worse yet, children with chronic pain or medical challenges are targets for teasing or bullying. The anxiety that accompanies this type of peer victimization not only is emotionally stressful, but also can significantly exacerbate pain conditions. In some situations peer-based difficulties are so stressful for kids that they can even be a root cause of a chronic pain condition.

Parents who have a child with pain often lament that their child is lonely, acts withdrawn, or is disinterested in seeing friends. Understanding the contributing factors of this problem and how to help scaffold a child's return to a healthy social life is a worthy goal that is often inextricably tied to the recovery from chronic pain. Whether your child was the popular kid on the soccer team, loved by everyone in the theater club, or enjoyed the quiet, comfortable company of a few close friends, it's important to think about how your child's pain and medical stress have changed the way he or she interacts with friends and other peers.

The disruption to peer relationships is usually related to both the physical and behavioral changes that go along with chronic pain. For example, kids may not be able physically to keep up with friends, may miss out on the day-to-day interactions at school, or may have to miss after-school activities due to pain or doctor appointments. Changes in memory, attention, or mood, too, may make him or her less patient with peers. Additionally, difficulties caused by chronic pain are not just hard to manage around peers; they are hard to explain.

Consider the difference between a child with a broken foot and one with chronic, neuropathic pain in a foot. With a broken bone, little explanation is needed. A child simply explains, "I broke my foot. I need to use crutches for three weeks and I can't play soccer for six weeks." Friends say, "Oh, that stinks." The child with the broken foot may be out of school for a day or two and feel frustrated to be off a soccer team temporarily, but generally understands that it will all be over soon and keeps a positive attitude about getting back on the team. Moreover, while there may be minor disruptions to activities, the child's friend group—and his or her place in it—won't change.

With neuropathic foot pain, by contrast, getting the right diagnosis may take several weeks, the severity of the pain and the ability to walk on the foot may wax and wane, and all the while the foot may look fine (that is, no cast or brace). Kids with neuropathic pain may use crutches one week and play at recess without them the next. In this more complex situation the suffering child often doesn't know what to say to friends. The variable nature of the symptoms creates a lot of confusion, and because peers may have no context for understanding the symptoms, they may even choose not to believe the child who is in pain. Even a hint of disbelief can cause kids with pain to avoid or limit activities or contacts with friends. All of these factors can wreak havoc with social connections.

Explaining Symptoms to Friends

In second grade my son suddenly started to hate getting his hair cut. When I asked what was going on, he explained that on the day after he gets a new haircut, his friends at school all comment on it the moment he walks into school. Did he get teased? No. They simply pointed out the haircut by saying, "Hey, you got a haircut" or "Nice haircut." These comments weren't negative in any way, but he hated this kind of attention. As a result, he fervently preferred to have his hair grow into his eyes and ears. The idea that he would avoid getting singled out at all costs highlights an important, albeit lamentable, aspect of some stages of child socialization; namely, being different feels like a problem. If getting a routine haircut can draw uncomfortable attention to a child in school, what must it be like to be a child with obvious chronic pain symptoms or pain-related supports?

Parents should not underestimate how anxious children can become when anticipating attention or questioning by their peers, especially when they don't have a clear medical or diagnostic explanation for their symptoms. "How can I explain this to my friends?" is one of the most frequent questions I am asked when I work one on one with kids in therapy. After acknowledging that this is a common and understandable problem, there are several important steps that need to be taken. First I work to make sure that a child has a developmentally appropriate understanding of his or her own symptoms or conditions. Next the child and I work together to clarify that most friends ask a lot of questions because they are naturally curious, not mean-spirited. Questions like "Where have you been?," "What's the matter with you?," "Why do you always go to the doctor?," "When are you going to get better?," or "Why can't you go to gym?" can feel harsh and accusatory, but it is important to let kids know that these questions, while perhaps not posed with great finesse, are not usually designed to make them feel bad. Instead, they should be thought of as an opportunity to connect with peers.

Almost all children struggling with chronic pain or medical illness are asked questions like these, and how they respond to them matters quite a lot. Fortunately, parents and kids can practice how to respond as a way of boosting confidence and helping kids feel prepared to return to school and other activities.

I strive to empower kids to share as much or as little as they want about their medical difficulties and their pain. If kids are uncomfortable discussing their situation with peers for any reason, they certainly should not feel pressured to do so. But there are advantages to opening up and talking about the situation to friends. For this reason, I often suggest that a child create a list of short responses to share with kids at school with whom they may not have close connections, and to develop a more detailed version of their medical- or pain-related challenges to share with their close friends. In our therapy session, we write these responses down and then practice them with a role play so that he or she can rehearse how the conversation might unfold. We focus not only on what a child says, but also on *how* the message is delivered.

Parents can easily do this with their child. If you're creative, working humor into this exercise can be helpful. Keep the responses age-appropriate, and work with your child to lower his or her guard by focusing on trying to connect with peers rather than being defensive about these questions. For example, when a peer asks, "Where have you been?" and a child responds, "None of your business," the conversation is over and the social connection is, at least temporarily, shut down. In contrast, consider some of the following examples:

"WHERE HAVE YOU BEEN?"

◆ Hey, thanks for asking. I've been sick, but I'm feeling better now.

◆ I've had the worst week. I had to go to see four different doctors. It's good to be back and not at the doctor today.

◆ I had some horrible headaches, but don't remind me. I'm glad to be back today.

◆ I was on a totally awesome vacation. What have you been up to?

"WHAT'S THE MATTER WITH YOU?"

◆ I know, it's crazy how much school I've missed. All I can say is I'm not contagious and I will get better—soon I hope.

◆ The bad news is that I keep getting really awful stomach pain; the good news is that it's not a horrible disease and eventually will go away.

◆ I have nerve pain. It's kind of a confusing condition, but I can explain it to you if you really want to know more.

"WHEN ARE YOU GOING TO GET BETTER?"

◆ That's a really good question. I hope soon. It stinks missing out on all the basketball games.

◆ I know, it feels like I've been sick forever. I'm glad to say I think things are already starting to improve.

◆ It's hard to say. My pain seems to come and go. It's really confusing to me so trust me; I'm not surprised that you're confused, too.

"WHY DO YOU MISS SO MUCH SCHOOL?"

◆ Yeah, I bet it seems like I get off easy. But when I'm not in school I'm either at the doctor, at physical therapy, or at home trying to catch up on work. It's not fun.

◆ Why? Are you looking for ideas for how to get out of school? Seriously, missing one or two days can be fun, but missing as much as I do makes it really hard to catch up.

♦ Mostly I miss school when I don't feel well. What I have is not like a cold or flu; my symptoms can come and go. So I miss a lot of school. It's really frustrating.

It's important that your child feels comfortable with an explanation, so be sure that whatever your child decides to say feels natural to her.

As for a longer explanation, this should also feel natural. Some kids like to print out educational material from the Internet for their friends or family or share materials that were given to them at the doctor's office. There are also some great websites that can be a helpful tool for explaining chronic pain conditions to peers (see Appendix 1). Interestingly, when kids with pain are in charge of explaining their condition to others, it can spur them to gain a greater command over it. In fact, if kids feel comfortable enough and motivated to do so, they might also consider giving a presentation to their class to explain their condition. I would never push a child to do this, but if kids are at ease talking to the class, this type of intervention can go a long way toward helping them to feel more comfortable with friends at school or in other settings.

Coping with Discomfort and Staying Connected

Talking to friends and explaining chronic pain is one hurdle; managing symptoms around friends is another. Amazingly, many kids with chronic pain and illness can cover up their symptoms almost entirely when they are at school. In fact, sometimes kids are such good actors that teachers and friends have little idea that they are suffering from pain or discomfort. I give these kids a lot of credit. It's exhausting to put on a good face every day and to not let anyone know that they are hurting. But some of these kids seem to pay the price at home when the school day ends. The backlash for covering up symptoms all day can take the form of physical or mental exhaustion, emotional upheaval, and at times, increased pain.

Yet while covering up symptoms can be challenging, the truth is that it's also rewarding and effective: "faking it" can actually help kids to be more functional. Consider that when kids are trying not to look bothered by symptoms, they are choosing to actively stay focused or engaged with other things. Yes it's hard to do, but if your child is faking it and getting through the day, that's a good sign that he or she is already accessing some good coping skills.

If your child is not coping well around friends, however, then help is needed. Kids often feel embarrassed or worried about having pain or medical symptoms in front of friends, so they need a few select strategies that they can use to help them mitigate discomfort and minimize negative peer attention. For example, for a child with back pain who is struggling to sit through class, using a subtle mindfulness strategy like focusing on tapping a five-word mantra on a table to distract the mind or engaging in deep breathing to relax the body is sometimes less obvious than standing up in class to stretch. If your child is worrying about how to cope with pain around friends, brainstorm together about strategies that won't leave him or her feeling alienated.

When a child is limited by pain or disability, it's important to think outside the box. For example, if a child is depressed that he or she can't play soccer for a season and misses his or her teammates, parents may be able to encourage or help facilitate their child's involvement in the team as a manager or assistant coach. The goal is to think of a way that your child might find a less time-consuming or physically demanding role as a short-term strategy for maintaining affiliation and engagement with important activities and peers. Staying connected to valued activities, whatever they might be for your child, is a proven way to maintain positive peer involvement and boost mood.

You may also consider offering alternative activities to your child. If she can't run on the soccer field, can she swim in a pool? If he can't commit to weekly debate club meetings, can he volunteer at a local animal shelter once a month? If she can't take Tae Kwon Do, can she do yoga? While the alternate activity may not be a first choice, encourage your child to take this opportunity to try something new and different. Perhaps your child will meet new friends in the process. Even better, perhaps your child can invite an old friend to join in the adventure of trying something new. Although taking things in a new direction can feel like defeat to some kids, remind your child that this new direction isn't about stalling out; it's a way to move forward.

Social Anxiety

Social anxiety or social phobia is the anxiety associated with being judged negatively by others. People with social anxiety have an intense fear that they will make mistakes, be embarrassed, or look bad in the eyes of others. This irrational fear is highly distressing for people and can cause panic attacks and even avoidance of social situations. Social anxiety is the third most common mental health illness and is associated with chronic pain conditions in adulthood. Perhaps not surprisingly, social anxiety usually flares for the first time during adolescence, a time when peer opinions are critical and self-identities are still in development. Kids with social anxiety typically feel upset when they perceive that others will be watching them or judging them in some way. For example, kids may fear being the center of attention, shy away from meeting new people, try to get out of giving a report in class, avoid talking on the telephone, or feel embarrassed about eating, drinking, or working in front of others. This anxiety can be so significant that it triggers the fight or flight response—the autonomic nervous system alarm that produces racing heart, shortness of breath, shaking, sweating, nausea, and upset stomach. Even anticipatory social anxiety such as worrying about an upcoming class presentation that isn't scheduled for three weeks can trigger panic in people with social anxiety.

Most people deal with anxiety, particularly social anxiety, with avoidance. In other words, when kids anticipate that they may be in a social situation in which others could potentially judge them in a negative way, they avoid going, which is something of a reward because it feels safe and comfortable. Avoidance means that there is no need for anxiety, at least in the short term—but it also means that kids miss learning that most of these feared social situations turn out just fine. Instead what they learn is that when they feel anxious, avoidance works well. This makes it more difficult for children to engage in the next social situation, leading to a cycle of increased social isolation and avoidance that is difficult to break.

Research shows that multiple factors contribute to the development of social anxiety. First, as with other anxiety disorders, there is a familial link. If other relatives in the family have an anxiety disorder, kids may have a biological vulnerability to social anxiety. Second, some research suggests that social anxiety may be linked to a dysregulation in the autonomic nervous system's fight or flight response. This is particularly salient for kids with pain since we know that pain can cause heightened arousal of the autonomic nervous system. Psychological or environmental factors can also contribute to the development of social anxiety. For example, children who have been bullied or have experienced an embarrassing social situation may be at increased risk for social anxiety. Additionally, kids who may not have age-congruent social skills may be primed to develop social anxiety.

When you consider the frequency with which social anxiety occurs, the role that the autonomic nervous system plays in the development of both chronic pain and social anxiety, the fact that social anxiety typically first becomes a problem in adolescence (not adulthood), and the likelihood that a child with chronic pain or illness has experienced a social situation that was perceived as embarrassing, it becomes worthwhile to evaluate if social anxiety could be causing or maintaining peer-based difficulties.

Fortunately, social anxiety is very treatable. Cognitive behavioral therapy is the gold-standard treatment, and there are several psychopharmacological medications that can also be helpful. If you suspect that your child has become socially anxious, even if it seems due to pain or medical stress, check in with a behavioral medicine provider, and do it sooner rather than later. The longer that social anxiety persists, the more alienated that kids become and the harder it is to get back on track.

Bullying

It's common for kids with pain to experience some disruption in their peer relationships. For a significant minority of children with chronic pain and medical difficulties, however, peer-based issues can be much more serious. Kids who are "different" can be targets for bullies, and even a child who has been popular and enjoyed positive friendships in the past might find that the symptoms of chronic pain trigger mean-spirited actions and remarks from peers.

The Centers for Disease Control and Prevention (CDC) defines bullying as any unwanted aggressive behavior that is repeated, or likely to be repeated, and that involves an observed, or perceived, power imbalance. Importantly, this power imbalance is not just about physical strength. A power imbalance can be related to popularity, physical ability, cognitive ability, or other factors. The effects of bullying can have serious and long-lasting effects on a child's mental health and daily functioning. Bullying can also interfere significantly with school attendance. Research shows that 15 percent of all school-related absences are a result either of bullying or of a fear of being bullied. Moreover, one in ten kids drop out of school altogether as a result of peer victimization. For these reasons, over the past several years bullying has drawn increased media attention and importantly, increased government regulation and oversight in the public school systems.

The incidence of bullying in schools within the United States is staggering. Bullying is most prevalent in middle schools, where approximately 30 to 35 percent of children ages eleven to fourteen report being bullied in school during the past school year. In high school, the incidence rate drops to approximately 20 to 25 percent. Of these cases, the vast majority (77 percent) involve verbal bullying, which can include teasing, rumor spreading, name-calling, sexual comments or gestures, or threatening. Other types of bullying involve physical victimization (pushing, hitting, shoving, or stealing personal items) and intentional social alienation or shunning. The incidence rates for bullying skyrocket for children with physical disabilities, learning difficulties, gender- or sexual-identity differences, or cultural differences. For example, 90 percent of kids who identify as being gay and 60 percent of kids with learning difficulties report having been bullied in school.

Cyber bullying, which is defined as any bullying that takes place online, has become a growing problem, though the current statistics on cyber bullying vary considerably. This variability is likely due to the newer nature of this type of peer victimization and the various forms it can take (text, Twitter, Instagram, email, Facebook, Foursquare, and so on). Some research suggests that as many as 80 percent of kids ages fourteen to eighteen have been bullied online. Other statistics find that cyber bullying is still far less common than in-school bullying, with incidence rates as low as 16 percent. Either way, parents need to consider that even if bullying is not an issue at school, bullies can still bother a child online.

Many parents think they would know if their child is being bullied either at school or online. But in 70 to 80 percent of cases, parents are not aware that their child has been bullied. It's easy for parents to gloss over the idea that their child may be the target of bullying, and no parent wants to think of their child suffering this type of social difficulty. So when kids deny that bullying is an issue, parents tend to breathe a sigh of relief and put the idea out of their minds. The problem is that kids are motivated to minimize or deny the social difficulties they are having. Kids may feel embarrassed or even blame themselves when they have been a target of bullying. Moreover, many kids worry that parent or school involvement will only make the situation worse. For these reasons, when I work with kids who are frequently absent from school or are avoiding peers, I routinely urge parents to go beyond asking their child if there is a problem. If school attendance is poor, or if a child avoids peer-based activities, parents should reach out to teachers, counselors, coaches, and parents of other kids at school to better understand how their child is doing socially. Parents may also need to monitor their child's social media to ascertain if cyber bullying may be a problem.

One of the most disheartening statistics on bullying is that in 85 percent of cases, the school does not intervene to support victims. Even when schools do get involved, if they are not knowledgeable about bullying interventions, they may approach the situation with mediation-based tactics that try to help the bully and the victim to resolve their issues. Unfortunately, mediation is proven not to work in these situations and can be traumatizing for the victim. It frequently takes parent advocacy to get the ball rolling in the right direction, though knowing how to be a good advocate for your child in this situation is often very challenging.

One resource for parents is the advice of Peter Raffali, a neurologist at Boston Children's Hospital who founded the Bullying and Cyberbullying Prevention and Advocacy Collaborative (BACPAC), the first of its kind in the country. It provides multidisciplinary evaluations with the aid of a neurologist, social worker, and educational specialist— evaluations that are then used to create a comprehensive plan to address bullying and support a child's social and emotional well-being at school. Raffali was inspired to start this clinic because so many of his neurology patients were being bullied at school and little was being done to properly rectify the problem. His recommendations are clear and firm: in cases of bullying, schools must step in to separate bullies from their victims. Of paramount importance is protecting the victim. Raffali stresses that bullying is never the victim's fault, and that it is critical that parents and schools communicate this directly to a child who has been victimized. While every state has its own legislation about bullying, parents should not hesitate to contact a local or state agency to learn more about how to intervene to support their child if they suspect that bullying is a problem and the school has not responded swiftly with appropriate action. Fortunately, there are many resources currently available to support parents and schools in this endeavor. There are several helpful websites listed at the end of this chapter.

The Overly Social Child

While loneliness, social anxiety, and peer victimization are commonly linked to chronic pain problems and persistent medical stress, sometimes I hear from parents and kids that kids seem to be too social. Having strong friendships that withstand the inherent stress of pain and illness is wonderful, but sometimes the scales tip too far in that direction. Some parents struggle because they report that their child appears too uncomfortable to go to school during the week, but then acts "fine" with friends on the weekends. It's certainly true that the positive influence of friends can be emotionally rewarding and mood boosting and can effectively distract kids from their pain or suffering. In fact, this is one of the reasons we emphasize the importance of kids staying closely connected to peers while they are coping with chronic pain. But when children are *only* well when their friends are around, parents should take note. For example, when kids don't miss an opportunity to walk through the mall shopping with girlfriends for two hours on Saturday, but report that they can't complete a fifteen-minute walk as part of a home exercise plan, there is clearly something amiss. Certainly a two-hour walk in the mall with friends is a great way to build in some daily exercise with the added bonus of positive peer support. But when kids function only when their friends are around or when peer activities are given higher priority than important goals such as completing make-up work for school or maintaining good sleep hygiene, parents may need to step in to set some limits. Sit down with your child and look over his or her schedule for the week. Be sure that your child has some opportunities for quality time with his or her friends during the week. If your child is able to get other essential areas of life on track, he or she could earn additional time with friends: a win-win for all.

Friends in All the Right Places

When children's school attendance and activities are disrupted, they may struggle to figure out how, when, and where to stay connected to peers. Often kids' first instinct is to keep their heads down and their computers or smartphones on around the clock. Certainly social media offers an easy opportunity to see what is going on in the lives of friends. In fact, the proliferation of social media means that kids can literally observe every minute of their friends' lives. This can be a great way to stay in the loop, but clearly social media is no substitute for face-to-face social connections and over time it can have a negative impact. When kids are constantly bombarded with images from events they missed or inside jokes they don't get, they may start to feel worse about their situation, not better. Moreover, exchanges over social media are often misconstrued and can unnecessarily complicate friendships. So while social media can be an effective tool for staying connected, it's certainly important to encourage kids to unplug and get some face-to-face time with friends.

Sometimes kids with pain or medical stress may find a welcoming community of peers in an illness-based support network. For example, the national arthritis and sickle cell foundations have active peer networks. If your child is struggling with a new diagnosis or has felt left out by friends who don't understand his or her medical issues, affiliation with a reputable organization that offers positive peer support can be very beneficial. But be careful: although kids like to connect with others who are struggling, and knowing they are not alone is enormously helpful to some children, when they become too aligned with an illness group the illness and disability can become a greater part of their identity. The goal for all kids is to learn how to cope with their symptoms and get back to a full and happy life. So if your child does connect with a pain or illness group, carefully monitor this involvement to ensure that the organization is reputable, that the connections are positive, and that the focus is on getting better, not on wallowing in pain or disability.

◆

How to Help

1. VALIDATE THE CHALLENGE OF STAYING CONNECTED TO PEERS

Parents are encouraged to talk openly with their kids about the challenges of staying connected and maintaining positive friendships in the midst of chronic pain and medical stress. This validation will go a long way toward helping your child begin the process of thinking about how to keep his or her social connections strong and how to react constructively to any problems.

2. PRACTICE WHAT TO SAY AND HOW TO SAY IT

Encourage your child to come up with responses and explanations for their pain or limited function that feel comfortable and natural.

Your child may want to have a few quick and easy responses for casual friends, and for closer friends, more in-depth ways of explaining or sharing their experiences. (Humor can help if it feels right, too.) Then practice using these responses and give your child feedback on how the message comes across. Be encouraging, and remind your child that the questions they hear will most commonly be asked out of simple curiosity.

3. MAKE A PLAN FOR COPING WITH DISCOMFORT

Kids will have more confidence in their ability to manage pain around friends when they know exactly what to do if their pain escalates while they are out of the house. Make a list of strategies that your child can use independently, and help your child to determine a plan for when he or she should seek adult support. Your child should actively participate in creating this list; if he or she feels that any strategy is likely to draw attention to the problem or be socially awkward in other ways, find an alternate approach.

4. CONSIDER THE ROLE OF SOCIAL ANXIETY

Social anxiety emerges in adolescence and an alienating experience such as chronic pain can definitely trigger it. A family history of social anxiety, or a child who tries to avoid a variety of social situations, should be red flags. Working with a cognitive behavioral therapist is key if you suspect that social anxiety is interfering with your child's ability to make and keep friends or interact successfully with peers.

5. KEEP AN EYE OUT FOR BULLYING

Bullying can occur without parents noticing. Physical, emotional, or behavioral differences can all increase the likelihood that a child will become a victim of bullying. If a child is avoiding school or social situations, parents should let her know that if she is being bullied, it's not her fault. Be clear with your child, too, that the situation may not resolve without adult intervention. Parents can also check in with other adults—teachers, parents, and coaches—who may have noticed how their child is doing socially. When school intervention is warranted, ensure that the tactic is separation, not mediation. You can check with state or local government agencies to learn more about how to protect your child if needed, and for more information on bullying see these helpful websites: www.thebullyproject.com, www.stopbullying.gov, or www.safeyouth.gov.

6. SET SOME BOUNDARIES IF NECESSARY

If your child is too active with friends and not attending to important recovery goals such as catching up on homework, exercising daily, or practicing good sleep hygiene, you should feel comfortable stepping in to set some boundaries. Friends are important, but not at the expense of keeping your child's recovery on track.

7. BE AWARE OF THE LIMITS OF ONLINE SOCIAL CONNECTIONS

While staying connected through social media can help to maintain connections with peers, and while online forums that welcome kids with similar medical illnesses or challenges can help your child feel less alone, there are potential downsides to these online connections. Social media comments can be misconstrued, and do not substitute for face-to-face conversations. Instead of always creating closeness, social media can actually further alienate your child and can complicate friendships. In addition, strongly identifying with one's pain or illness has been linked to increased disability from that pain or illness. So monitor your child's involvement in any online health-related networks to make sure that the messages are positive and that the goal of getting back into the flow of life is a main focus.

19
Family Matters

I run my chronic pain workshop, called the Comfort Ability, every six weeks at Boston Children's Hospital. The program is for children suffering from chronic pain and their parents. While the program provides much needed support to parents and kids, it's also arguably missing an important element. One of the most frequent questions we get during our enrollment for the program is "Can a sibling come too?" This question highlights one of the most challenging aspects of chronic pain, illness, and medical stress: namely, that they affect the whole family. It's not hard to list some of the myriad ways that a child's chronic pain can change family dynamics. Parents might miss work to stay home with a child, family vacations and activities may be put on hold, siblings may feel neglected and jealous, there may be more marital stress between parents, and routine day-to-day family activities can all be curtailed by a child's pain.

While it may be reassuring to know that these family disruptions commonly occur, most parents want to know how to reduce the impact of this situation on the family, for everyone's sake. Indeed, conflict and stress in the home environment are known triggers for increased pain-related disability in children with a wide range of underlying medical conditions. Importantly, the opposite can also be true; when families report cohesive relationships and lower levels of stress, pain and disability may be less impairing.

Investing in the care of the whole family when a child has chronic pain or stress is hard to do. It's easier to think "I'll deal with everything else later, let me just get through this crisis first." Unfortunately, this approach can cause more damage to family relationships down the road. It is vitally important to take the time to purposefully foster supportive, meaningful relationships between partners, between children and parents, and between siblings, and to nurture the family as a whole. When families are strong and healthy, they truly can be a safe haven during a time of stress.

Take Time to Reflect

You may remember from Chapter 4 that one of the best first strategies for helping children with pain to reduce their own feelings of negativity and frustration is to validate their experience. This validation is part of a strategy that is called "reflective listening." When you are engaging in reflective listening, you first give the person speaking a few moments of undivided attention during which you listen—really listen—to the problem, and then you respond by echoing what you think that person is likely experiencing emotionally or physically. When I teach this strategy to parents, I use the following example:

> Imagine that you come home from work after a long, hard day and your partner greets you at the door. Your partner can tell you are not yourself and asks, "What's wrong?" You jump at the chance to tell your partner about how your boss has unrealistic expectations and yelled at you for not completing an end-of-the-month report on time, even though she clearly prioritized the completion of other projects just yesterday. Now imagine that your partner replies: "Yeah, but if it was the end of the month, I can

understand why your boss would want the end-of-the-month report completed." You can probably feel your blood pressure rise. Whether your partner is right or wrong makes no difference in this scenario. What matters is that this was clearly not the answer you were looking for, and it has left you feeling angry and alone. Now imagine that your partner says, "Your boss is way out of line. She has no idea how hard you work every day to meet all of her ridiculous deadlines!" Ahh. Suddenly you are so glad to be home where you know people really and truly understand and support you.

When a family is under stress from having a child with pain or another medical problem, many family members may feel the fallout. For example, siblings may complain that no one cares about them, and partners may feel neglected. When a sibling says, "You never do anything for me," it's easy for parents to deny this statement with a quick "Of course that's not true." But if you are really taking time to connect, you might try responding, "I hear you. It seems that we are paying a lot of attention to your sister right now." Or if a partner is frustrated that there hasn't been a chance to eat a quiet meal or go on a date, it's easy to say, "I can't deal with that right now, I'm at my wits' end." But it doesn't take much more effort to reflect, "I also wish we had more quiet time in our lives right now; this is really hard." These powerful reflective statements get at the heart of the problem and go a long way toward helping family members connect with each other, even if there is no quick solution to the problem at hand.

Importantly, a reflective statement can also often open the door for a constructive conversation about how to manage a family-based challenge. For example, if parents can't go out to dinner for a date, perhaps a jointly scheduled coffee break or even a ten-minute walk through the neighborhood can be part of the interim solution. Once you've validated a family member's feelings, it's far easier to work together to find a solution. Taking an extra minute or two to use a reflective listening approach is a fool-proof strategy for helping to maintain cohesiveness at home. Don't hold back—try using it with siblings, partners, and even extended family members. The simple power of heartfelt reflective listening will amaze you.

Caring for Siblings

For the past thirty years, research on how siblings fare when a child in the family has a chronic medical condition has been divided. One branch of the research suggests that siblings are an "at-risk" population that is more vulnerable to anxiety, depression, acting-out behaviors, lower self-esteem, and other psychosocial difficulties. The other branch, by contrast, suggests that these siblings are perhaps more resilient than their peers. The rationale is that siblings of a child with pain or illness might adapt by taking on a more mature or independent role in the family. Moreover, it's been suggested that the act of caring for a sick sibling may lead to more compassionate sibling relationships.

In 2002 a meta-analysis evaluated the outcomes of fifty studies to try to draw some conclusions from the murky research in this field. This study concluded that siblings of children with chronic illness are slightly more at risk for emotional or behavioral difficulties as compared to kids who had healthy siblings, but not by much, and interestingly, the type or severity of a sibling's illness did not alter the findings. What was a significant variable, however, was the day-to-day impact these symptoms had on the family; the more a child's symptoms disrupted the family relationships and activities, the more significant the risk for siblings. The good news for parents, then, is that the overall impact on siblings is pretty small and can be countered.

It's vitally important that parents don't expect that a sibling will have consistent compassion for a child in the family who has ongoing pain. Of course siblings feel bad for the child with discomfort, but when the symptoms or medical involvement starts to take a front seat in the family and all other matters (particularly theirs) get brushed aside, it's impossible for them not to feel slighted. While many siblings are vocal about this imbalance in the family, many other siblings don't complain much at all. They quietly harbor these feelings because admitting them makes them feel guilty. For this reason, it's more common for siblings to struggle with an internalizing disorder such as anxiety or depression instead of acting out. Whether a sibling is vocal or quiet about these challenges, parents should recognize and validate the inherent struggle. Just a few minutes of time each day dedicated to connecting with your children who are not experiencing pain can make an enormous difference. Try using reflective statements like

"I can see that the last few weeks have been really challenging for you."

"It seems to me that we've been pretty focused on your brother lately. I'm sure you're feeling that too."

"I can only imagine how stressful this is for you. I want you to know that I recognize the toll that this situation is taking on everyone."

"You must feel sometimes that no one even cares about your life anymore. It's been so hard to find time to connect with you with all the stress we've had around helping your sister."

As powerful as these reflective statements can be, it's important for parents to match their sincere words with meaningful action. I routinely suggest that parents build in what is called "non-contingent" child time. This is a great strategy to use with all children in the family. Here's the setup: parents tell each child that they'd like to reserve a little time each day, perhaps fifteen to thirty minutes, to just be together with no interruptions. The time can be spent playing a sport, talking, reading something together, or doing a simple activity like playing a board game or painting fingernails or toenails. (I advocate against screen-based activities for this intervention.) Importantly, the child should be in charge of deciding which activity occurs—in other words, parents shouldn't plan or guide the selection of the activity. Parents are encouraged to set a timer and make sure that during this protected time no interruptions occur.

This technique is termed "non-contingent" time because the intervention should not be contingent on anything. In other words, it doesn't matter if your child was good or bad that day, if they got an "A" or an "F" on a test at school, or if they did or did not complete their chores. The time occurs because it's important to the welfare of your child to have dedicated time to connect.

This dedicated time is always a good idea, but is especially important during times of family stress, when ideally it will be scheduled at least five days per week. This is why it's so important for parents to stick to a time limit that will be compatible with busy schedules and competing demands for parent time. If parents regularly extend their protected non-contingent time, kids will come to expect the additional time and then feel upset when they perceive that their time has been cut short. Parents should keep in mind that this time isn't set aside to discuss homework, chores, pain, or other potential problem areas: the goal is to develop protected time for positive parent-child interactions. Positive interactions hopefully are already happening throughout the day: a quick hug, a chat in the car, encouragement for work on a school project. But an additional fifteen minutes or so of quality time can truly enrich a parent-child connection and can be restorative for a sibling who can't help but feel the effects of the stress that comes along with having a brother or sister in pain.

Your child (especially an older adolescent) may find this intervention a little strange at first if you haven't had quality time alone for awhile. But give it a chance and keep at it for a few weeks. Soon kids start to crave this time, and even though parents sometimes doubt that it will be valuable, I truly cannot count the number of times that parents have thanked me for prescribing this strategy. As it turns out, parents come to enjoy and look forward to this quiet, protected time in the day as much as their children do. If there are two parents in the household, parents can either take turns or develop their own dedicated-time ritual with each child. It's a great way to foster positive relationships within the family.

Beyond the real (or perceived) lack of parent attention that is felt by so many siblings, there can be a general sense of injustice among siblings within the family. Some of the imbalance is clearly unavoidable.

For example, kids with chronic pain or medical issues may be physically unable to complete assigned chores, may need priority seating on the couch or in the car, may require special meals, and may determine when or if friends can visit. Yet there are still ways that parents can help to make the situation fair. For example, if a sibling has to pick up extra chores around the house to help out, figure out a plan for reciprocity or for showing that sibling appreciation. If a child in pain used to be responsible for emptying the dishwasher, but now can't easily do that task, figure out something that the child in pain can do for the sibling (for example, fold her laundry, help with homework) or a special way that you can reward the sibling who is putting forth extra effort. Involve all children in the family in developing a plan for reciprocity to ensure that everyone feels included and their concerns have been heard.

Reintegrating the Child with Pain

A child with pain or medical difficulties may occupy a somewhat unique role within the family environment. As part of my initial assessment with families, I always ask kids (while their parents are in the room), "What chores do you do at home?" Sometimes they rattle off a few tasks such as keeping their room clean or emptying the dishwasher, but the overwhelming majority of the time, kids look a little squirrelly when I ask this question. Their sideways glance to the parent tells me that they have somehow cheated the system. Parents may interject, "Well, he used to do chores, but now with all the doctor appointments and make-up work, there just isn't time." I don't think kids ever feign a disability for the sole purpose of getting out of family responsibilities. But it's not a bad perk.

As you think about supporting, or "scaffolding," your child's return to a more regular lifestyle, remember that part of this recovery involves your home and family life. Moreover, being helpful to others can mitigate feelings of helplessness, a challenge for many children with pain, stress, or disability. Finding ways to give back to the family can help the family function more smoothly, and when children are held accountable for doing chores around the house and contributing to family life, they have higher levels of self-efficacy—in other words, they feel more empowered and self-confident. Research shows that this self-efficacy often translates into a strong work ethic and greater success in adulthood. The daily and sometimes mundane chores that are necessary to keep a family going offer an excellent opportunity for kids of all ages to build important life skills; letting kids off the hook when it comes to chores may seem like a kind thing to do, but it doesn't serve kids well in the long run.

Just like for other goals, parents and kids should work together and start small when thinking about how to contribute to family life. With your child's particular challenges in mind, brainstorm ways that he or she can be useful to the family. For example, small chores around the house such as watering the plants, unpacking groceries, or sorting toys for donation can be done without much time or physical effort. If your child is more impaired, chores that can be done on a computer such as planning a menu of dinners for the week along with accompanying grocery lists, or researching a family outing or vacation, may be a good starting place.

Beyond initiating or maintaining chores, children with pain or illness should participate in family routines as much as possible. If everyone sits down together as a family for dinner, your child with pain should be expected to join, even if at first that means being at the table for only a limited amount of time. Similarly, if the family routine involves turning off the TV after 9:00 p.m., your child with pain should adhere to this as well. While there will undoubtedly be times when a child with pain will need to veer from family routines, the default expectation should be that the child with pain will stick to the family rules and actively contribute to the well-being of the group.

The Importance of the Partner Relationship

Having a child with chronic pain or illness is a significant source of stress in a committed relationship. Perhaps not surprisingly, research finds that this is a chicken-and-egg scenario. Having a child with chronic pain or medical stress places stress on a relationship, and a stressed relationship or conflict between partners can contribute to more entrenched pain and disability for a child. One study found that this connection holds true even when looking at a single health behavior such as sleep. In other words, kids who don't sleep are a source of stress for partners, and stress between partners can also be a root cause of poor sleep for kids. Given that kids with persistent pain and medical difficulties usually have many disrupted health behaviors, the potential for strain in a relationship is magnified.

One basic but persistent source of stress for many parents who have a child with pain or other medical difficulties is figuring out how to present a united front when addressing a child's symptoms. In many families, the parents have different styles of interacting with the children. For example, one parent may have a softer, more empathic approach and the other may be more matter-of-fact in his or her parenting approach. For more than fifty years, researchers in the field of developmental psychology have tried to identify exactly which parenting styles or practices promote healthy and well-adjusted children. Because there is now widespread recognition that multiple factors—including cultural, geographic, religious, and socioeconomic differences—influence parenting practices, there is not a single agreed-on standard. Yet it does seem that when parents are unified in their approach, are responsive to their child's needs, and jointly adhere to parenting practices that emphasize the value of attaining clear and reasonable expectations, kids respond.

As you may remember from the discussion in Chapter 1, we do know that overly protective parenting practices may unwittingly influence children to be less active and may also be linked to mood difficulties and increased anxiety. In contrast, when parents encourage activity and adaptive coping strategies, kids are more likely to be active and to have less associated disability. One of the keys to success is getting both parents to agree on a unified approach. It's hard to make progress when one parent adopts these ideas and works to hold their child accountable for working toward a more active recovery, but the other parent encourages rest or is overly protective.

I once worked closely with a Mom and her twelve-year-old daughter to help them manage a pain-related disability that was interfering with school and other activities. We set up activity and school attendance goals using the scaffolding techniques, set rewards for success, and mapped out how we were going to make small but incremental progress over the course of several weeks. I worked closely with the Mom in treatment and we seemed to be on the same page. Unfortunately, since the Dad's work schedule was very demanding, I never met him. About four weeks into our treatment, when we were exploring possible reasons why this child wasn't making the anticipated progress, I learned that the Dad was a gentle, kind man who was just a little too soft-hearted to stick to the plan. He struggled to hold his daughter accountable for her goals, and he gave her rewards when she hadn't met all of the criteria for earning them. Without a doubt his intentions were good; he was clearly trying to provide extra support and some special care to his struggling daughter. But the fallout was significant. The child lacked motivation in part because she knew her father would allow her to earn her prize regardless of whether or not she fully achieved her goals. Equally as important, the Dad's behavior undermined the Mom's efforts at home and left the Mom feeling alienated and angry. The Mom felt as though her husband was increasingly becoming the favorite parent while she had to be the "bad guy" who was forcing her child to do things that were emotionally and physically challenging. To address this issue, the Mom and Dad were both invited to a parent training session. First, we validated the Dad's desire to make his daughter feel better at any cost. We acknowledged that his behavior was an attempt to make his daughter feel special and loved, and not at all intended to alienate his wife. I emphasized that a big part of helping his daughter to feel better was to teach her that she could meet these important health-related goals. Once the Mom and Dad were on the same page with the plan, their daughter started to get back on track and make progress toward her recovery.

There are many ways that parents can work together to foster a collaborative partnership and to reduce stress. For example, while both parents have to remain knowledgeable about identified goals, in some instances it can work well to have parents be responsible for different aspects of a pain-management plan (for example, the Dad could be responsible for increasing the child's activity or exercise while the Mom takes on the job of school advocacy). In order for this to work, parents must communicate regularly about the goals and any progress. Sometimes the use of a shared notebook or log sheet can be a good way to communicate information between parents. When parents are working together in this way, the burden feels lighter and kids are more likely to succeed.

If there is ongoing stress between partners, the first thing to do is to discuss what's not working. Do parents have different approaches to taking care of a child with pain? Does one parent feel overburdened or burned out with day-to-day tasks? Has there been too little time to focus on each other? Discuss what might improve if changes could be made and set out to make some adjustments. If you are moving forward with changes, be sure to reconnect within a week to see how the modifications are going. Often new plans or approaches need tweaking along the way.

Parent Self-Care

Beyond taking time to care for siblings and partners, parents must take time to care for themselves. Parenting a child with chronic pain or medical stress is not easy. The research is unequivocal on this front. There are the challenges of managing all of the daily tasks involved with keeping a child with pain active, involved in school, and engaged with activities. Additionally, parents must support their child's emotional and physical well-being and keep the family intact. This is a tall order. While most parents can find the energy and fortitude to manage these challenges for weeks at a time, eventually this stress takes its toll. Numerous studies have documented that parents who care for a child with a chronic medical condition have more psychological distress, more relationship stress, and more dissatisfaction with life. In one study that assessed a group of parents who had a child with chronic pain, a full 66 percent of parents reported high stress. Beyond stress, parents whose children have chronic medical issues are also at risk for emotional burnout; 60 percent of parents reported clinical levels of anxiety and 40 percent reported depression.

While the majority of parents report that they have close relationships with their medically involved children, most parents candidly describe their child as being "difficult." The idea that parenting a child with pain is "difficult" is no doubt an understatement. It is easy to understand how a chronic condition can create chronic stress in the lives of parents. And this is not an indication of weakness or failure. To the contrary, I think these findings show that parents put every ounce of energy and time into helping their child and so have little time for self-care.

When I talk with parents about the need for self-care I have learned that simply encouraging parents to take some much needed respite so they will feel happier and healthier leads to few changes. I can only gain some traction when I share that when they are not caring for their own emotional or physical needs they are not at their best to care for their child. It's not uncommon for parents—both Moms and Dads—to quietly shed tears when we discuss this in session. Parental guilt, frustration, and feelings of inadequacy can feel crushing. I imagine that parents who have a child with a persistent medical condition might have these feelings many times over the course of weeks or months or even years. When a child is not thriving for any reason, parents feel desperately worried and responsible. I don't think we can undo this universal experience of parenting concern and guilt. But I do know from both my clinical and personal experiences that when parents take the time and energy to take care of themselves, the negative feelings are easier to manage. Less anxiety, depression, and stress means that parents can be more present and more helpful to their child. In contrast, continuing to harbor these negative feelings never makes the situation better.

Think of the management of chronic pain like a marathon, not a sprint. When training for a marathon you have to attend to many factors like diet, sleep, hydration, and physical training. During the marathon itself, you have to pace yourself, take water breaks, and generally follow your body's cues to let you know how fast and far you should be pushing yourself. If you forget one of those factors, or if you don't listen to your body, it can be hard to finish the race. When parents take breaks from the stress and get support for any mood-based difficulties, they are more equipped to finish the marathon. In contrast, when parents don't take time to care for themselves it's as if they forgot to eat the night before the big race; they simply run out of fuel. Parents instead should think of self-care as a part of the scaffolding that can support their child. Without this important piece in place it's hard for kids and parents to make progress in the recovery from chronic pain.

When parents are first trying to focus more on self-care, I strongly suggest that they schedule the time they need into their daily calendar and make it as non-negotiable as other important events, such as a scheduled medical appointment. Think about what has worked best for you during times of stress in the past and fall back on these favorite methods. Keep in mind, too, that the coping strategies reviewed in this book work equally well for parents and have the added benefit of modeling a healthy coping strategy for your child. For example, exercise is always a good strategy for de-stressing and the relaxation strategies reviewed in Part 3 can be adapted for parent use. Beyond these strategies, parents are encouraged to try other self-care approaches such as going out to lunch or dinner with supportive family and friends, taking a new class, picking up an old hobby, getting a massage, playing music, or journaling, to name just a few ideas.

Parents with Pain

Chronic pain can run in families. There are undoubtedly biological reasons for this association. Parents and kids share 50 percent of their genes and many medical conditions that are associated with chronic pain have a heritable component. But that is only one piece of the puzzle.

There is also a social learning component to pain. Factors such as how a parent thinks about his or her pain condition, and whether the parent chooses to attend to pain symptoms or ignore them, seem to influence how kids respond to their own pain symptoms. The modeling of pain-response behaviors strongly influences how well children and adolescents function in young adulthood and beyond. Parents who have their own pain conditions should try their best to model adaptive and active approaches to managing their own symptoms. Not only will this help to reduce a parent's personal struggle with pain and function, but also this positive modeling can be protective for children; parents who model adaptive coping with pain may reduce the likelihood that their children will struggle with persistent pain and disability in their adult lives.

When parents have their own pain, they clearly have a unique perspective into their child's pain. For example, endometriosis, a chronic pelvic pain condition that occurs in women, has a strong familial link, so mothers and adolescent daughters often share this diagnosis. Other conditions such as arthritis and migraine headache also run in families. Sharing a pain condition has the potential to be helpful; parents may have targeted ideas about what adaptive strategies or interventions may help their child based on their own success in managing symptoms.

Sometimes, though, when parents and kids share a pain problem, it's more challenging than helpful. Some parents adopt an "I just deal with it" attitude and thus view their child's struggle with pain or any pain-related disability as a sign of weakness. This approach can leave a child with pain feeling alienated and misunderstood. Other parents may identify too closely with their child who has pain and become overly attentive and concerned about their child's symptoms. If parents themselves have been unable to work, have become deconditioned from pain, or have had to forgo important family, work, or social obligations due to pain, they may expect their child will need to do the same. This thinking can undermine a child's sense that he can learn to cope with pain and so seriously hinder his recovery.

If you are a parent dealing with your own chronic pain, it's best not to assume that a child's experience is similar. Pain is an entirely subjective experience and even when parents and kids share the same diagnoses, the experience of pain and related disability can vary widely. Moreover, for children and adolescents, the course for chronic pain is even more variable. Thus while current estimates suggest that about one-third of kids with chronic pain will also have pain as adults, the majority—two-thirds—will not. Even for the kids who have chronic pain conditions that persist into adulthood, the level of impairment may vary. Many factors can positively or negatively influence these outcomes and parents may unintentionally do an injustice to their child when they assume that their child's experience will mirror their own.

◆

How to Help

1. USE REFLECTIVE LISTENING

The "reflective listening" strategy pairs undivided listening attention with empathic reflective statements. It's easy to do and it can work wonders for reducing feelings of irritability, sadness, stress, or other negative emotions in all members of the family. Parents are encouraged to use this valuable life skill often, with each other, with their child who has pain, and with his or her siblings.

2. PROVIDE SIBLING SUPPORT

Whether or not there is an obvious problem, siblings are at risk for emotional and psychosocial difficulties when there is a child with chronic pain or medical illness in the family. It's helpful for parents to openly address this issue with siblings and take action to rectify perceived imbalances in the family when possible. If siblings continue to struggle, you'll want to consider psychological support; ask your child's pediatrician for a referral.

3. ENCOURAGE YOUR CHILD TO BE AN ACTIVE FAMILY MEMBER

Children with pain may necessarily function somewhat differently within the family. Finding creative ways to help your child with pain give back to the family and adhere to family rules as much as possible, however, reinforces the important message that everyone in the family is expected to work together. For this reason, you and your child should be sure to add "participation in family activities and responsibilities" to the blueprint for recovery.

4. CARE FOR YOUR PARTNER

Having a child with chronic pain is inherently stressful, and this can place additional strain on a relationship. Additionally, conflict or stress within a relationship can translate to more stress and more pain for children. Making time for partners and ensuring that both partners are supporting each other not only promotes feelings of well-being in a relationship, but also can translate to happier and healthier children.

5. CO-PARENTING IS KEY

Little progress in the recovery from pain or pain-related disability can be made when two partners disagree on how to approach and manage the situation. If discussing problems, sharing ideas, and dividing responsibilities aren't helping, parents should consider a parenting consultation with a behavioral medicine provider.

6. CARE FOR YOURSELF

One reason that self-care is vitally important is that it models adaptive coping with stress. When you show (instead of just tell) your child how you take the time to actively reduce your own stress by going for a walk, having lunch with a friend, or taking quiet time to meditate, your child may be more likely to adopt these positive behaviors as well. The bonus, of course, is that you will feel better and have more stamina for managing the myriad challenges that arise when managing a child with chronic pain or other medical stress.

7. PARENTS WITH PAIN PLAY AN IMPORTANT ROLE

Pain is transmitted through genetics and through observable behaviors. In other words, it has elements of both nature and nurture. If you are a parent with pain it's important to remember that your child will learn how to cope with his or her own symptoms in part by watching you. Adopting helpful coping skills and active approaches to pain management will help you both to feel better. Moreover, even when you share the same diagnosis as your child, the experience of pain can vary significantly. Remain positive and stay focused on the idea that a significant majority of children with pain do learn how to function better.

8. CONSIDER FAMILY OR COUPLES COUNSELING

Many of the family-based disruptions that commonly occur are hard to repair without support. Families who are struggling to meet the challenges of managing a child's ongoing pain, disability, or medical stress are routinely encouraged to seek additional support for their relationships with partners and family because happy, healthy family relationships can most definitely help children's recovery. The American Association for Marriage and Family Therapy (AAMFT) has a referral website that can help you to locate a qualified provider in your area; see www.therapistlocator.net.

Part V

Recommended Resources

The following resource guide was developed in conjunction with the goals of this book—to provide up-to-date access to information that is demonstrated to be helpful in the management of a child's ongoing pain and pain-related stress. While this book reviews many important topics, additional or more in-depth understanding of various problems is often warranted. The materials listed in this section should help parents looking for additional information on topics related to their child's experience.

The websites listed in Appendix 1 may be useful resources for parents, but are also excellent ways to share information with your child, with siblings, or with other family members or friends. Most children or adolescents will look online for information about pain and other health-related topics. Showing them websites that have targeted and accurate information can be an important intervention and may minimize the likelihood of their consuming inaccurate or misleading information online. Additionally, if you're thinking about exploring a new intervention with your child, such as acupuncture or behavioral medicine, reading about it online and listening to others share a first-hand account of the intervention may help parents and kids alike to have a better understanding of what to expect.

The book and video recommendations in Appendix 2 include resources for parents and children. There are many pain-related materials, but this list also includes numerous resources for managing stress, fear, and anxiety in children. There are two reasons for this. First, recall that chronic pain creates an enormous amount of stress in the lives of children. So accruing additional strategies beyond the scope of this book for managing stress, fear, and anxiety can be very helpful. Second, many of the cognitive and behavioral strategies that are used to manage stress, fear, and anxiety in children—such as relaxation-based skills and the use of exposure-based principles to increase function (that is, doing a little bit at a time to gain confidence)—parallel the strategies used for the management of chronic pain. So even if your child is not struggling with fear or anxiety, many of the resources listed for anxiety may be useful for reinforcing the cognitive behavioral strategies for pain that have been introduced in this book.

The list of apps in Appendix 3 came about from a systematic review that my colleagues and I conducted to identify apps that included pain-management content and empirically supported skills, were easy for kids to use, and used an engaging interface. This list of annotated apps is divided into categories to help parents and children select those that may be best suited for their particular needs. But parents should keep in mind that the technology is constantly advancing and the availability of any given app is subject to change at any time, so this list cannot be considered comprehensive. Additionally, these apps were all tested on an Apple operating system, and although many are also available on other operating systems (Android, Samsung), availability varies by app. When shopping for apps, be wary: while apps may be a useful tool for reinforcing pain-management skills, apps not on this list may not have been developed in conjunction with pain-management professionals and may not represent best practice parameters.

Appendix 4 contains a list of pediatric pain-management programs by state as published by the American Pain Society. This list, updated every two years, includes programs that incorporate multi-disciplinary and interdisciplinary services and encompasses outpatient, day-treatment, and inpatient facilities. If your child has been struggling with chronic pain, has not made progress with the strategies in this book, and has not yet had a comprehensive evaluation by a pediatric pain management program, it can be worthwhile to call the program nearest to you and inquire about the process for evaluation and treatment. While the nearest program may still be quite far from where you live, pain management programs, often after an initial evaluation, can refer children to providers within their home communities and continue to monitor progress with intermittent visits. Additionally, an evaluation in a comprehensive pain management program can help to determine what level of care may be best for your child's needs. Outpatient services are typically recommended as a first line treatment. But there are also intensive programs (day-treatment and inpatient) that are designed especially for children and adolescents who have a high level of disability associated with their pain and have not responded to targeted outpatient services. Notably, many of the websites listed in this appendix may serve the dual purposes of helping to identify the closest pain management center and being a valued resource with targeted information about chronic pain management. With chronic pediatric pain now recognized as one of the most costly pediatric problems, new pediatric pain management centers and resources are in a state of rapid development. As such, parents should keep in mind that additional resources may be available beyond those listed in the table.

Helpful Websites

General Pediatric Health Information

American Academy of Pediatrics
http://www.healthychildren.org
Informative resource addressing a wide range of topics and issues in pediatric healthcare including healthy sleep habits, good nutrition, sports and fitness recommendations, and emotional wellness.

Kids Health from Nemours
http://kidshealth.org/parent
Website with parent information and resources regarding a variety of pediatric conditions.

For More on Pediatric Pain

Pain and Your Child or Teen
http://www.med.umich.edu/yourchild/topics/pain.htm
Terrific resource from the University of Michigan Health System that explains how pain works in the body and reviews pain medications.

Pain Resource Centre
http://www.aboutkidshealth.ca/En/ResourceCentres/Pain/Pages
/default.aspx
Helpful guide for general information about pediatric pain.

Child-Friendly Health Information

Kids Health from Nemours
http://kidshealth.org/kid, http://kidshealth.org/teen
These interactive websites provide helpful and targeted information to kids
and teens regarding a variety of health-related issues.

Integrative Medicine
http://chc.remotocom.com/CIM
A great series of videos featuring children talking about acupuncture, biofeedback, hypnosis, aromatherapy, and massage.

Pain Bytes
http://www.aci.health.nsw.gov.au/chronic-pain/painbytes
Comprehensive resource for learning about pain and behaviorally based
pain-management skills. Includes engaging videos of children and families
talking about pain management and charts to track progress.

School Resource on Pediatric Pain

Teach Pain
https://teachpain.wordpress.com
Informational website for teachers and school staff regarding chronic pain.
Can also be helpful for interested family and friends.

For Assistance in Locating Providers in the United States

Academy of Nutrition and Dietetics
http://www.eatright.org/programs/rdnfinder
This website offers a search area for finding a licensed dietitian/nutritionist
(LDN) for your child.

American Association for Marriage and Family Therapy

http://www.therapistlocator.net

This referral website from the AAMFT will help you to locate a qualified provider of marriage and family therapy near you.

American Psychological Association

The public education information line of the American Psychological Association, 1-800-964-2000, can be a good place to start when looking for a behavioral medicine provider.

Association for Behavioral and Cognitive Therapists

http://www.abct.org

Clicking on the "find a CBT provider" link on this helpful website will pull up a search tool that will allow you to access a list of behavioral and cognitive therapists in your area.

Biofeedback Certification International Alliance

http://www.bcia.org

To identify a local provider who is board certified in biofeedback, parents can log on to this website and click on the "Find a Practitioner" link.

Move Forward PT

http://www.moveforwardpt.com

The official American Physical Therapy Association website offers a wealth of information for patients, including recommended providers.

Useful Books and Videos

Parenting Books That Address Pain

Butler, David. 2013. *Explain Pain,* 2d ed. Adelaide, Aust.: NOI Group.

Diamond, S., and A. Diamond. 2010. *Headache and Your Child: The Complete Guide to Understanding and Treating Migraine and Other Headaches in Children and Adolescents.* New York: Simon and Schuster.

Krane, E. J. 2007. *Relieve Your Child's Chronic Pain: A Doctor's Program for Easing Headaches, Abdominal Pain, Fibromyalgia, Juvenile Rheumatoid Arthritis, and More.* New York: Simon and Schuster.

Levy, J. 2004. *My Tummy Hurts: A Complete Guide to Understanding and Treating Your Child's Stomachaches.* New York: Simon and Schuster.

Olivia-Hemker, M., D. Ziring, and A. Bousvaros. 2010. *Your Child with Inflammatory Bowel Disease: A Family Guide for Caregiving.* Baltimore: The Johns Hopkins University Press.

Zeltzer, L. K., and C. B. Schlank. 2005. *Conquering Your Child's Chronic Pain: A Pediatrician's Guide for Reclaiming a Normal Childhood.* New York: Harper Collins Living.

Parenting Books That Address Child Stress and Anxiety

Chansky, T. 2004. *Freeing Your Child from Anxiety: Powerful, Practical Solutions to Overcome Your Child's Fears, Worries, and Phobias.* New York: Three Rivers Press.

Greenland, S. K. 2010. *The Mindful Child.* New York: Free Press.

Pincus, D. B. 2012. *Growing Up Brave: Expert Strategies for Helping Your Child Overcome Fear, Stress, and Anxiety.* Lebanon, IN: Hachette Digital.

Rapee, R. M., et al. 2008. *Helping Your Anxious Child: A Step-by-Step Guide for Parents.* Oakland, CA: New Harbinger.

Child Books for Managing Stress (Ages 6 to 11)

Crist, J. J. 2004. *What to Do When You're Scared or Worried: A Guide for Kids.* Minneapolis: Free Spirit.

Huebner, D., and B. Matthews. 2005. *What to Do When You Worry Too Much: A Kid's Guide to Overcoming Anxiety (What to Do Guides for Kids).* Self-published by D. Huebner.

Shapiro, L. E., and R. K. Sprague. 2009. *The Relaxation and Stress Reduction Workbook for Kids: Help for Children to Cope with Stress, Anxiety and Transitions.* Oakland, CA: New Harbinger.

Adolescent Books for Managing Stress (Ages 12 to 17)

Fox, M. G., and L. Sokol. 2011. *Think Confident, Be Confident for Teens: A Cognitive Therapy Guide to Overcoming Self-Doubt and Creating Unshakeable Self-Esteem.* Oakland, CA: New Harbinger.

Schab, L. M. 2008. *The Anxiety Workbook for Teens: Activities to Help You Deal with Anxiety and Worry.* Oakland, CA: New Harbinger.

Tompkins, M., and K. Martinez. 2010. *My Anxious Mind: A Teen's Guide to Managing Anxiety and Panic.* Washington D.C.: Magination Press.

Parenting Books That Discuss School Function

Kearney, C. 2007. *Getting Your Child to Say "Yes" to School.* New York: Oxford University Press.

Mayer, D. P. 2008. *Overcoming School Anxiety: How to Help Your Child Deal with Separation, Tests, Homework, Bullies, Math Phobia, and Other Worries.* New York: American Management Association.

Videos about Pain for Parents and Adolescents

"The Mystery of Chronic Pain" A TED Talk by Dr. Eliot Krane.
   http://www.ted.com/talks/elliot_krane_the_mystery_of_chronic_pain.
   An interesting talk about how chronic pain works and how to treat it.
   Includes a real-life patient example.
"Why Things Hurt." A TED Talk by Dr. Lorimer Moseley.
   http://tedxtalks.ted.com/video/TEDx-Adelaide-Lorimer-Moseley-W.
   An informational talk about how the brain is involved in the experience
   of pain.

Innovative Apps for Pain
Management and Relaxation

Below are some great apps for guiding your child's experiences with pain management and relaxation. For more background on the survey that resulted in this list, see the 2015 paper by K. Smith, C. Iversen, J. Kossowsky, S. O'Dell, R. Gambhir, and R. Coakley, titled "Apple Apps for the Management of Pediatric Pain and Pain-Related Stress," in *Clinical Practice in Pediatric Psychology*, 3 (2), 93–107.

General Meditation and Relaxation

◆ Autogenic Training and Progressive Muscle Relaxation—$2.99. This app has an educational focus throughout, and includes an explanation of every exercise. The exercises, each of which is less than 15 minutes long, include muscle relaxation, autogenic training, breathing meditation, and imagery. 01 Digitales Design GmbH, 2012.

◆ Cleveland Clinic Stress Meditations—$0.99. This app is better suited for older adolescents. The app includes a good selection of meditations, each of which includes helpful educational information about the benefits of relaxation before each exercise. Cleveland Clinic Wellness Enterprise, 2012.

◆ Relax and Rest Guided Meditations—$0.99. This easy-to-use guided meditation app has three different lengths of meditation, and both the voice and background music are very soothing. The longest meditation (24 minutes) has components of muscle relaxation, which may be particularly helpful for pain. Other meditations focus on breath (5 minutes) and deep rest (13 minutes). Meditation Oasis, 2011.

◆ Simply Being: Guided Meditation for Relaxation and Presence—$0.99. This app is designed for adults but is one of the highest-rated meditation apps in the App Store and would work well for adolescents. Meditations have several different lengths, so adolescents could work up to the longer meditations. Emphasis is on "letting go" and "just being." Meditation Oasis, 2009.

Diaphragmatic ("Belly") Breathing

◆ Breathe2Relax—Free. This app teaches people how to belly breathe. It includes instruction and a single practice exercise. This app is especially helpful for pacing one's breathing and the practice screen is very customizable. The National Center for Telehealth and Technology, 2011.

◆ Pranayama—Free. This breathing app is based on principles of breathing in yogic practice. This guide to deep breathing has a progressive course that includes music and animated visuals. Saagara, 2011.

Pain Management

◆ Healing Buddies Comfort Kit—$4.99. This application is best for children under age 12. It incorporates several different biobehavioral exercises, including relaxation, imagery, acupressure, and aromatherapy. The voice can be either male or female, and both are very soothing. This app also includes a parent segment. Designwise Medical, 2013.

◆ Pain Tricks—Free. This app has a lot of great information for parents and some good information for younger children. It includes examples and information about pain, distraction techniques, relaxation, and breathing, though it does not incorporate much practice. Cilein Kearns, 2012.

General Cognitive Behavioral Therapy

◆ Anxiety Coach—$4.99. This app has great information about anxiety, but it may be too text-heavy or complicated for young children; adolescents are more likely to find it useful. The app tries to provide guidance on exposure-based principles of anxiety reduction, but can be confusing to navigate. Mayo Clinic, 2012.

♦ At Ease: Anxiety and Worry Relief—$2.99. This app has three different guided breathing meditations, each from nine to twelve minutes long, that are designed to reduce anxiety. This app also features support for technical difficulties, and a journaling component that allows users to keep track of "inner resources." Meditation Oasis, 2010.

♦ CBT Tools for Kids—$1.99. This application is designed by a psychologist and is good for most ages. It contains excellent relaxation exercises. It is also designed to supplement CBT. It includes a strong cognitive component and could be useful for children and parents to do together. Veronica Cregg, 2013.

♦ CBT4Kids Toolbox—Free. This app is designed by psychologists for children ages six to twelve. It is to be used in conjunction with therapy and is very user-friendly and good for beginners. This application features a breathing game and a progressive muscle relaxation exercise, and the user can buy more modules within the app. CBT4Kids; A Henry & LL Kokkoris, 2013.

♦ eCBT Mood—$0.99. This application is best for adolescents. It has a strong educational focus regarding what CBT is and its potential benefits, and it includes an optional password. This app's strong cognitive component includes a thought log, thought identification tool, thought challenging tool, and mood assessments. The user can also set a medication reminder. Mind-Apps LLC, 2012.

♦ Take a Chill—Stressed Teens—$1.99. This app is good for teenagers who are stressed, especially about school. It includes exercises that target test anxiety and thought stopping. Users can track their progress over time. It also includes reminders to engage in practice. Channel Capital, LLC, 2012.

Sleep

♦ iSleep Easy Meditations for Restful Sleep—$4.99. This app has nine different meditations that focus on initiation of sleep. It also includes a good meditation to be used for middle of the night awakenings. These meditations vary in length from 2 to 15 minutes and include education and practice for diaphragmatic breathing and autogenic relaxation. Meditation Oasis, 2012.

◆ Sleep Well!—$3.00. This app has child-friendly education incorporated into it, and a soothing voice (male or female) to calm listeners. The app is simple and straightforward and incorporates deep breathing into every exercise. Each exercise is 6 to 10 minutes long. Somatiq, LLC, 2015.

Yoga

◆ My Five-Minute Yoga Practice—$2.99. This app has several different short (just five minutes long) routines that target different body parts and incorporate various stretches. It also includes longer yoga sessions—some of which are premade and others that allow the user to combine different shorter modules for a customized routine. The app is very user-friendly for adolescents, but the model in the video is an older woman, which may not appeal as much to teens. Eve Johnson, 2011.

◆ Super Stretch Yoga—Free. This app was created as a story led by a super-hero that kids follow through different yoga poses. This app is good for very young children. Parents and children can use this app together. The Adventures of Super Stretch, LLC, 2001.

Pain-Management Programs, by State

State	City	Name of Program	URL
AR	Little Rock	Pediatric Pain Medicine, Arkansas Children's Hospital	http://www.archildrens .org/Services/Pediatric -Pain-Management.aspx
AZ	Phoenix	Pediatric Pain Service, Phoenix Children's Hospital	http://www.phoenix childrens.com
CA	Irvine	UC Irvine Healthcare Center for Pain Manage-ment, UC Irvine Douglas Hospital	http://www.anesthesiology .uci.edu/pain
CA	Los Angeles	Pediatric Pain Manage-ment Clinic, Children's Hospital Los Angeles	http://www.chla.org/ site/c.ipINKTOAJsG/ b.4991943/k.81B0/ Chronic_Pain.htm

State	City	Name of Program	URL
CA	Los Angeles	UCLA Pediatric Pain Program—Pediatric Pain Clinic & Whole Child LA, David Geffen School of Medicine at UCLA	http://www.mattel.medsch .ucla.edu/pedspaina.org http://www.wholechildla .org
CA	Palo Alto	Pediatric Pain Management Service–Chronic Pain Management Clinic, Lucile Packard Children's Hospital at Stanford	http://pedsanesthesia .stanford.edu/patient _care/pain.html
CA	San Francisco	Pediatric Integrative Pain Clinic, University of San Francisco Children's Hospital	http://www.osher .ucsf.edu/patient-care/ treatments-services/ pediatrics-2/pediatrics
CO	Aurora	Pain Consultation Services, Children's Hospital Colorado	http://www.childrens colorado.org/ (no website: Chronic outpatient #720-777-6700)
CT	Hartford	Division of Pain Medicine: Chronic Pain Program, Connecticut Children's Medical Center	http://www.connecticut childrens.org/our-care/ pain-and-palliative -medicine
DC	Washington	Complex Pain Management Center, Children's National Medical Center/ Sheikh Zayed Institute for Pediatric Surgical Innovation	http://childrensnational .org/departments/pain -medicine-care-complex
DE	Wilmington	Integrated Pain and Wellness Program, Nemours/ Alfred I. DuPont Hospital for Children	http://www.nemours.org/ service/medical/pain management.html

State	City	Name of Program	URL
GA	Atlanta	Center for Pain Relief, Children's Healthcare of Atlanta	http://www.choa.org/ childrens-hospital-services/ pain-relief
IL	Chicago	Chronic Pain Management Program, Ann and Robert H. Lurie Children's Hospital of Chicago	https://www.luriechildrens .org/en-us/care-services/ specialties-services/ anesthesiology/chronic -pain-treatment/Pages/ index.aspx
IL	Chicago	RIC Center for Pain Management, Rehabilitation Institute of Chicago	http://www.ric.org/ paincenter
KY	Louisville	Children's Health and Illness Recovery Program (CHIRP)–Kosair Children's Hospital and Bingham Clinic, University of Louisville School of Medicine Pediatrics Child Psychiatry and Psychology	http://louisville.edu/chirp
MA	Boston	Pediatric Chronic Pain Program, Boston Children's Hospital	http://www.childrens hospital.org/clinical services/Site1897/main pageS1897P0.html
MA	Waltham	Mayo Pediatric Pain Rehabilitation Center, Boston Children's Hospital at Waltham	http://www.childrens hospital.org/clinical services/Site2585/main pageS2585P0.html
MA	Waltham	Pediatric Chronic Headache Program, Boston Children's Hospital at Waltham	http://www.childrens hospital.org/clinical services/Site2589/main pageS2589P0.html

State	City	Name of Program	URL
MD	Baltimore	Pediatric Pain Rehabilitation Program, Kennedy Krieger Institute	http://www.childrensdmc.org/?id=1814&sid=1
MI	Detroit	Children's Hospital of Michigan Pediatric Pain Management Program	http://www.childrensdmc.org/?id=1814&sid=1
MN	Minneapolis	Interdisciplinary Pain Clinic, Children's Hospitals and Clinics of Minnesota	http://www.childrensmn.org/services/pain-program
MN	Rochester	Pediatric Chronic Pain Clinic, Mayo Clinic	http://www.mayoclinic.org/pain-medicine-rst
MO	Kansas City	Abdominal Pain Program, Children's Mercy Hospitals and Clinics	http://www.childrensmercy.org/abpain
MO	Kansas City	Comprehensive Pain Management Clinic, Children's Mercy Hospitals and Clinics	http://www.childrensmercy.org/Clinics_and_Services/Clinics_and_Departments/Pain_Management
MO	St. Louis	St. Louis Children's Hospital Pain Management Clinic, St. Louis Children's Hospital	http://www.stlouischildrens.org/our-services/pain-management-clinic
NJ	New Brunswick	Pediatric Chronic Pain Center, Children's Specialized Hospital	http://www.childrens-specialized.org/Programs-Services/Inpatient-Programs/Pain-Management.aspx

State	City	Name of Program	URL
NY	New York	Pediatric Pain Management Center, Morgan-Stanley Children's Hospital of New York	http://childrensnyp.org/mschony/pain-medicine.html
OH	Cincinnati	Pain Management Clinic, Cincinnati Children's Hospital Medical Center	http://www.cincinnatichildrens.org/svc/alpha/p/pain/default.htm
OH	Cleveland	Pediatric Pain Rehabilitation Program, Cleveland Clinic Children's Hospital	http://my.clevelandclinic.org/childrens_hospital/departments/rehabilitation_services/programs/pediatric_pain_rehab.aspx
OH	Columbus	Comprehensive Pain Services, Nationwide Children's Hospital	http://www.nationwidechildrens.org/pain-service-clinic
OH	Dublin	Center for Pediatric and Adolescent Pain Care, Private Practice	http://www.pediatricpaincare.com
OK	Oklahoma City	Pediatric Pain Management, The Children's Hospital at OU Medical Center	http://www.oumedicine.com/body.cfm?id=6427
OR	Portland	Pediatric Pain Management Center, OHSU Doernbecher Children's Hospital	http://www.ohsu.edu/xd/health/services/doernbecher/programs-services/pain-management.cfm
PA	Hershey	Pediatric Chronic Pain Clinic, Penn State Milton S. Hershey Medical Center	http://www.pennstatehershey.org/web/anesthesia/patientcare/services/pediatric-chronicpain

State	City	Name of Program	URL
PA	Philadelphia	Pain Management Program, Children's Hospital of Philadelphia (CHOP)	http://www.chop.edu/service/painmanagementprogram/
TX	Dallas	Pediatric Pain Management Center, Children's Medical Center	http://www.childrens.com/specialties/pain-management
TX	Fort Worth	Pediatric Pain Management Program, Cook Children's Hospital	http://www.cookchildrens.org/SpecialtyServices/Pain%20Management/Pages/default.aspx
WA	Seattle	Pain Medicine Program, Seattle Children's Hospital	http://www.seattlechildrens.org/clinics-programs/pain-medicine
WI	Milwaukee	Jane B. Pettit Pain and Palliative Care Center–Chronic Pain Clinic, Children's Hospital of Wisconsin, Medical College of Wisconsin	http://www.chw.org/medical-care/pain-management-program

Source: "Pediatric Chronic Pain Programs by State," available online at the American Pain Society's website: http://americanpainsociety.org/uploads/get-involved/Pediatric PainClinicList_Update_2.10.15.pdf (accessed April 28, 2015).

References and Suggested Reading

Part I. On Your Mark

Evans, S., et al. 2010. "Sociodemographic Factors in a Pediatric Chronic Pain Clinic: The Roles of Age, Sex, and Minority Status in Pain and Health Characteristics." *Journal of Pain Management* 3 (3): 273–281.

Haraldstad, K., et al. 2011. "Pain in Children and Adolescents: Prevalence, Impact on Daily Life, and Parents' Perception—A School Survey." *Scandinavian Journal of Caring Sciences* 25 (1): 27–36.

Howard, R. F. 2003. "Current Status of Pain Management in Children." *JAMA* 290 (18): 2464–2469.

Konijnenberg, A. Y., et al. 2004. "Children with Unexplained Pain: Do Pediatricians Agree Regarding the Diagnostic Approach and Presumed Primary Cause?" *Pediatrics* 114 (5): 1220–1226.

Lier, R., T. Nilsen, and P. Mork. 2014. "Parental Chronic Pain in Relation to Chronic Pain in Their Adult Offspring: Family-Linkage within the HUNT Study, Norway." *BMC Public Health* 14: 797.

Lindley, K. J., D. Glaser, and P. J. Milla. 2005. "Consumerism in Healthcare Can Be Detrimental to Child Health: Lessons from Children with Functional Abdominal Pain." *Archives of Disease in Childhood* 90 (4): 335–337.

Mazurek, M. O., et al. 2013. "Anxiety, Sensory Over-Responsivity, and Gastro-intestinal Problems in Children with Autism Spectrum Disorders." *Journal of Abnormal Child Psychology* 41 (1): 165–176.

Chapter 1. Beyond Intuition

Claar, Robyn Lewis, Laura E. Simons, and Deirdre E. Logan. 2008. "Parental Response to Children's Pain: The Moderating Impact of Children's Emotional Distress on Symptoms and Disability." *Pain* 138 (1): 172–179.

Eccleston, C., et al. 2012. "Psychological Interventions for Parents of Children and Adolescents with Chronic Illness." Review. *Cochrane Collaboration* 8: 1–109.

Evans, S., et al. 2010. "Associations between Parent and Child Pain and Functioning in a Pediatric Chronic Pain Sample: A Mixed Methods Approach." *International Journal on Disability and Human Development* 9 (1): 11–21.

Fales, J. L., et al. 2014. "When Helping Hurts: Miscarried Helping in Families of Youth with Chronic Pain." *Journal of Pediatric Psychology* 39 (4): 427–437.

Garwick, A. W., et al. 1998. "Parents' Perceptions of Helpful vs. Unhelpful Types of Support in Managing the Care of Preadolescents with Chronic Conditions." *Archives of Pediatrics and Adolescent Medicine* 152 (7): 665–671.

Langer, S. L., et al. 2009. "Catastrophizing and Parental Response to Child Symptom Complaints." *Child Health Care* 38 (3): 169–184.

Simons, Laura E., Robyn Lewis Claar, and Deirdre L. Logan. 2008. "Chronic Pain in Adolescence: Parental Responses, Adolescent Coping, and Their Impact on Adolescents' Pain Behaviors." *Journal of Pediatric Psychology* 33 (8): 894–904.

von Baeyer, C. L. 2009. "Numerical Rating Scale for Self-Report of Pain Intensity in Children and Adolescents: Recent Progress and Further Questions." *European Journal of Pain* 13 (10): 1005–1007.

Chapter 2. The Science of Pain and the Mind-Body Connection

Apkarian, A. V. 2010. *Human Brain Imaging Studies of Chronic Pain: Translational Opportunities. Translational Pain Research: From Mouse to Man.* Edited by L. Kruger and A. R. Light. Boca Raton, FL: Taylor and Francis.

Berryman, C., et al. 2013. "Evidence for Working Memory Deficits in Chronic Pain: A Systematic Review and Meta-Analysis." *Pain* 154 (8): 1181–1196.

Butler, David. 2013. *Explain Pain,* 2d ed. Adelaide, Aust.: NOI Group.

Coakley, R. M., and N. L. Schechter. 2013. "Chronic Pain Is Like . . . : The Clinical Use of Analogy and Metaphor in the Treatment of Chronic Pain in Children." *Pediatric Pain Letter* 15 (1): 1–8.

Colloca, Luana, et al. 2013. "Placebo Analgesia: Psychological and Neurobiological Mechanisms." *Pain* 154 (4): 511–514.

Crettaz, Benjamin, et al. 2013. "Stress-Induced Allodynia—Evidence of Increased Pain Sensitivity in Healthy Humans and Patients with Chronic Pain after Experimentally Induced Psychosocial Stress." *PLoS One* 8 (8).

Griffin, Sarah C., and Jack W. Tsao. 2014. "A Mechanism-Based Classification of Phantom Limb Pain." *Pain* 155 (11): 2236–2242.

Landrø, Nils Inge, et al. 2013. "The Extent of Neurocognitive Dysfunction in a Multidisciplinary Pain Centre Population: Is There a Relation between Reported and Tested Neuropsychological Functioning?" *Pain* 154 (7): 972–977.

Latremoliere, A., and C. J. Woolf. 2009. "Central Sensitization: A Generator of Pain Hypersensitivity by Central Neural Plasticity." *Journal of Pain* 10 (9): 895–926.

Moriarty, Orla, Brian E. McGuire, and David P. Finn. 2011. "The Effect of Pain on Cognitive Function: A Review of Clinical and Preclinical Research." *Progress in Neurobiology* 93 (3): 385–404.

Park, S. H., and R. H. Mattson. 2009. "Ornamental Indoor Plants in Hospital Rooms Enhanced Health Outcomes of Patients Recovering from Surgery." *Journal of Alternative and Complementary Medicine* 15 (9): 975–980.

Rideout, Victoria J., Ulla G. Foehr, and Donald F. Roberts, 2010. "Generation M2: Media in the Lives of 8- to 18-Year-Olds." Rep. Menlo Park: Henry J. Kaiser Family Foundation.

Schwenkreis, P., C. Maier, and M. Tegenthoff. 2009. "Functional Imaging of Central Nervous System Involvement in Complex Regional Pain Syndrome." *American Journal of Neuroradiology* 30 (7): 1279–1284.

Simons, L. E., I. Elman, and D. Borsook. 2014. "Psychological Processing in Chronic Pain: A Neural Systems Approach." *Neuroscience and Biobehavioral Reviews* 39: 61–78.

Tajerian, M., et al. 2014. "Brain Neuroplastic Changes Accompany Anxiety and Memory Deficits in a Model of Complex Regional Pain Syndrome." *Anesthesiology* 121 (4): 852–865.

Ursin, H. 2014. "Brain Sensitization to External and Internal Stimuli." *Psychoneuroendocrinology* 42: 134–145.

Woolf, Clifford J. 2011. "Central Sensitization: Implications for the Diagnosis and Treatment of Pain." *Pain* 152 (supp. 3): S2–S15.

Chapter 3. The Unavoidable Link between Pain and Stress

Anda, R., et al. 2010. "Adverse Childhood Experiences and Frequent Headaches in Adults." *Headache* 50 (9): 1473–1481.

Anderberg, U. M., et al. 2000. "The Impact of Life Events in Female Patients with Fibromyalgia and in Female Healthy Controls." *European Psychiatry* 15 (5): 295–301.

Andress-Rothrock, D., W. King, and J. Rothrock. 2010. "An Analysis of Migraine Triggers in a Clinic-Based Population." *Headache* 50 (8): 1366–1370.

Bonilla, S., and M. Saps. 2013. "Early Life Events Predispose the Onset of Childhood Functional Gastrointestinal Disorders." *Revista de Gastroenterología de México* 78 (2): 82–91.

Centers for Disease Control and Prevention. 2012. "Youth Risk Behavior Surveillance—United States, 2011," MMWR 61, no. SS-66104, pp. 1–168. Available at http://www.cdc.gov/mmwr/preview/mmwrhtml/ss6104a1 .htm (accessed April 25, 2015).

Cohen, L. L., K. E. Vowles, and C. Eccleston. 2010. The Impact of Adolescent Chronic Pain on Functioning: Disentangling the Complex Role of Anxiety. *Journal of Pain* 11 (11): 1039–1046.

Crettaz, Benjamin, et al. 2013. "Stress-Induced Allodynia—Evidence of Increased Pain Sensitivity in Healthy Humans and Patients with Chronic Pain after Experimentally Induced Psychosocial Stress." *PLoS One* 8 (8).

Leeuw, M., et al. 2007. "The Fear-Avoidance Model of Musculoskeletal Pain: Current State of Scientific Evidence." *Journal of Behavioral Medicine* 30 (1): 77–94.

Miller, G. E., E. Chen, and K. J. Parker. 2011. "Psychological Stress in Childhood and Susceptibility to the Chronic Diseases of Aging: Moving toward a Model of Behavioral and Biological Mechanisms." *Psychology Bulletin* 137 (6): 959–997.

Simons, L. E., and K. J. Kaczynski. 2012. "The Fear Avoidance Model of Chronic Pain: Examination for Pediatric Application." *Journal of Pain* 13 (9): 827–835.

Simons, Laura E., et al. 2012. "Fear of Pain in the Context of Intensive Pain Rehabilitation among Children and Adolescents with Neuropathic Pain: Associations with Treatment Response." *Journal of Pain* 13 (12): 1151–1161.

Chapter 4. Managing Negativity, Frustration, and Doubt

Burbach, Daniel J., and Lizette Peterson. 1986. "Children's Concepts of Physical Illness: A Review and Critique of the Cognitive-Developmental Literature." *Health Psychology* 5 (3): 307–325.

Claar, Robyn Lewis, Laura E. Simons, and Deirdre E. Logan. 2008. "Parental Response to Children's Pain: The Moderating Impact of Children's Emotional Distress on Symptoms and Disability." *Pain* 138 (1): 172–179.

Eccleston, Christopher, et al. 2004. "Adolescent Chronic Pain: Patterns and Predictors of Emotional Distress in Adolescents with Chronic Pain and Their Parents." *Pain* 108 (3): 221–229.

Hechler, T., et al. 2011. "Parental Catastrophizing about Their Child's Chronic Pain: Are Mothers and Fathers Different?" *European Journal of Pain* 15 (5): 515 e1–9.

Kalish, C. 1996. "Causes and Symptoms in Preschoolers' Conceptions of Illness." *Child Development* 67 (4): 1647–1670.

Williamson, Gail M., Andrew S. Walters, and David R. Shaffer. 2002. "Caregiver Models of Self and Others, Coping, and Depression: Predictors of Depression in Children with Chronic Pain." *Health Psychology* 21 (4): 405–410.

Chapter 5. Redefining Comfort

Karoly, P., and L. S. Ruehlman. 2006. "Psychological 'Resilience' and Its Correlates in Chronic Pain: Findings from a National Community Sample." *Pain* 123 (1–2): 90–97.

Kilic, S. A., D. S. Dorstyn, and N. G. Guiver. 2013. "Examining Factors that Contribute to the Process of Resilience Following Spinal Cord Injury." *Spinal Cord* 51 (7): 553–557.

Newton-John, T. R., C. Mason, and M. Hunter. 2014. "The Role of Resilience in Adjustment and Coping with Chronic Pain." *Rehabilitation Psychology* 59 (3): 360–365.

Stewart, D. E., and T. Yuen. 2011. "A Systematic Review of Resilience in the Physically Ill." *Psychosomatics* 52 (3): 199–209.

Sturgeon, J. A., and A. J. Zautra. 2010. "Resilience: A New Paradigm for Adaptation to Chronic Pain." *Current Pain and Headache Reports* 14 (2): 105–112.

Chapter 6. Behavioral Medicine

Barakat, Lamia P., Elizabeth R. Gonzalez, and Beverley Slome Weinberger. 2007. "Using Cognitive-Behavior Group Therapy with Chronic Medical Illness." In *Handbook of Cognitive-Behavior Group Therapy with Children and Adolescents: Specific Settings and Presenting Problems,* edited by R. W. Christner, J. L. Stewart, and A. Freeman. New York: Routledge.

Beck, A. T. 1979. *Cognitive Therapy and the Emotional Disorders.* New York: Meridian.

Crosby, L. E., et al. 2012. "Integrating Interactive Web-Based Technology to Assess Adherence and Clinical Outcomes in Pediatric Sickle Cell Disease." *Anemia* 2012: 492428.

Eccleston, C., et al. 2002. "Systematic Review of Randomised Controlled Trials of Psychological Therapy for Chronic Pain in Children and Adolescents, with a Subset Meta-Analysis of Pain Relief." *Pain* 99 (1–2): 157–165.

———. 2012. "Psychological Interventions for Parents of Children and Adolescents with Chronic Illness." Review. *Cochrane Collaboration* (8): 1–109.

Grewal, S., M. Petter, and A. Feinstein. 2012. "The Use of Distraction, Acceptance, and Mindfulness-Based Techniques in the Treatment of Pediatric Pain." *Pediatric Pain Letter* 14 (1): 1–9.

Hayutin, L. G., et al. 2009. "Skills-Based Group Intervention for Adolescent Girls with Inflammatory Bowel Disease." *Clinical Case Studies* 8 (5): 355–365.

Hofmann, S. G., et al. 2012. "The Efficacy of Cognitive Behavioral Therapy: A Review of Meta-analyses." *Cognitive Therapy and Research* 36 (5): 427–440.

Kendall, P.C. 2012. "Guiding Theory for Therapy with Children and Adolescents." In *Child and Adolescent Therapy: Cognitive-Behavioral Procedures,* edited by P. C. Kendall. New York: Guilford Press.

Knook, Lidewij M. E., et al. 2011. "Psychiatric Disorders in Children and Adolescents Presenting with Unexplained Chronic Pain: What Is the Prevalence and Clinical Relevancy?" *European Child and Adolescent Psychiatry* 20 (1): 39–48.

Lackner, J. M., et al. 2008. "Self-Administered Cognitive Behavior Therapy for Moderate to Severe Irritable Bowel Syndrome: Clinical Efficacy, Tolerability, Feasibility." *Clinical Gastroenterology and Hepatology* 6 (8): 899–906.

Law, E. F., et al. 2014. "Systematic Review and Meta-Analysis: Parent and Family-Based Interventions for Children and Adolescents with Chronic Medical Conditions." *Journal of Pediatric Psychology* 39 (8): 866–886.

Logan, Deirdre E., and Laura E. Simons. 2010. "Development of a Group Intervention to Improve School Functioning in Adolescents with Chronic Pain and Depressive Symptoms: A Study of Feasibility and Preliminary Efficacy." *Journal of Pediatric Psychology* 35 (8): 823–836.

McCracken, Lance M. 2005. *Contextual Cognitive-Behavioral Therapy for Chronic Pain.* Seattle: IASP Press.

Morrison, Norma. 2001. "Group Cognitive Therapy: Treatment of Choice or Sub-Optimal Option?" *Behavioural and Cognitive Psychotherapy* 29 (3): 311–332.

Palermo, T. M. 2009. "Enhancing Daily Functioning with Exposure and Acceptance Strategies: An Important Stride in the Development of Psychological Therapies for Pediatric Chronic Pain." *Pain* 141 (3): 189–190.

Palermo, T. M., et al. 2009. "Randomized Controlled Trial of an Internet-Delivered Family Cognitive-Behavioral Therapy Intervention for Children and Adolescents with Chronic Pain." *Pain* 146 (1–2): 205–213.

Palermo, Tonya M., Cecelia R. Valrie, and Cynthia W. Karlson. 2014. "Family and Parent Influences on Pediatric Chronic Pain: A Developmental Perspective." *American Psychologist* 69 (2): 142–152.

Rogers, R. 2008. *Managing Persistent Pain in Adolescents.* Oxford: Radcliffe Publishing.

Stinson, J., et al. 2009. "A Systematic Review of Internet-Based Self-Management Interventions for Youth with Health Conditions." *Journal of Pediatric Psychology* 34 (5): 495–510.

Wetherell, J. L., et al. 2011. "A Randomized, Controlled Trial of Acceptance and Commitment Therapy and Cognitive-Behavioral Therapy for Chronic Pain." *Pain* 152 (9): 2098–2107.

Weydert, J. A., et al. 2006. "Evaluation of Guided Imagery as Treatment for Recurrent Abdominal Pain in Children: A Randomized Controlled Trial." *BMC Pediatrics* 6: 29.

Wicksell, R. K., et al. 2009. "Evaluating the Effectiveness of Exposure and Acceptance Strategies to Improve Functioning and Quality of Life in Long-standing Pediatric Pain—A Randomized Controlled Trial." *Pain* 141 (3): 248–257.

Yovel, I. 2009. "Acceptance and Commitment Therapy and the New Generation of Cognitive Behavioral Treatments." *Israel Journal of Psychiatry and Related Sciences* 46 (4): 304–309.

Chapter 7: Physical and Occupational Therapy

Ayling Campos, A., et al. 2011. "Clinical Impact and Evidence Base for Physiotherapy in Treating Childhood Chronic Pain." *Physiotherapy Canada* 63 (1): 21–33.

Bowering, K. J., et al. 2013. "The Effects of Graded Motor Imagery and Its Components on Chronic Pain: A Systematic Review and Meta-Analysis." *Journal of Pain* 14 (1): 3–13.

Deconinck, F. J., et al. 2014. "Reflections on Mirror Therapy: A Systematic Review of the Effect of Mirror Visual Feedback on the Brain." *Neurorehabilitation and Neural Repair,* pp. 1–13.

Hoffart, C. M., and D. P. Wallace. 2014. "Amplified Pain Syndromes in Children: Treatment and New Insights into Disease Pathogenesis." *Current Opinion in Rheumatology* 26 (5): 592–603.

Holsti, L., C. Backman, and J. Engel. 2013. "Occupational Therapy." In *Oxford Textbook of Paediatric Pain,* edited by P. A. McGrath et al. Oxford, Eng.: Oxford University Press.

Jamieson-Lega, K., R. Berry, and C. A. Brown. 2013. "Pacing: A Concept Analysis of the Chronic Pain Intervention." *Pain Research and Management* 18 (4): 207–213.

Johnson, M. I., C. H. Ashton, and J. W. Thompson. 1991. "An In-Depth Study of Long-Term Users of Transcutaneous Electrical Nerve Stimulation (TENS): Implications for Clinical Use of TENS." *Pain* 44 (3): 221–229.

Moseley, G. L., A. Gallace, and C. Spence. 2008. "Is Mirror Therapy All It Is Cracked Up to Be? Current Evidence and Future Directions." *Pain* 138 (1): 7–10.

Tupper, et al. 2013. "Physical Therapy Interventions for Pain in Childhood and Adolescence." In *Oxford Textbook of Paediatric Pain,* edited by P. A. McGrath et al. Oxford, Eng.: Oxford University Press.

Chapter 8. Medications and Supplements

Argoff, C. E. 2013. "Topical Analgesics in the Management of Acute and Chronic Pain." *Mayo Clinical Proceedings* 88 (2): 195–205. doi: 10.1016/j.mayocp.2012.11.015.

Bailey, J. E., E. Campagna, and R. C. Dart. 2009. "The Underrecognized Toll of Prescription Opioid Abuse on Young Children." *Annals of Emergency Medicine* 53 (4): 419–424. doi: 10.1016/j.annemergmed.2008.07.015.

Charrois, T. L., et al. 2006. "Peppermint Oil." *Pediatric Review* 27 (7): e49–e51.

Derry, S., et al. 2014. "Topical Lidocaine for Neuropathic Pain in Adults." *Cochrane Database Systematic Reviews* no. 7: Cd010958. doi: 10.1002/14651858.CD010958.pub2.

Diener, H. C., et al. 2005. "Efficacy and Safety of 6.25 mg t.i.d. Feverfew CO2-extract (MIG-99) in Migraine Prevention—A Randomized, Double-Blind, Multicentre, Placebo-Controlled Study." *Cephalalgia* 25 (11): 1031–1041. doi: 10.1111/j.1468–2982.2005.00950.x.

Gibbons, R. D., et al. 2010. "Gabapentin and Suicide Attempts." *Pharmacoepidemiology and Drug Safety* 19 (12): 1241–1247. doi: 10.1002/pds.2036.

Jick, H., J. A. Kaye, and S. S. Jick. 2004. "Antidepressants and the Risk of Suicidal Behaviors." *JAMA* 292 (3): 338–343. doi: 10.1001/jama.292.3.338.

Kaminski, A., et al. 2011. "Antidepressants for the Treatment of Abdominal Pain-Related Functional Gastrointestinal Disorders in Children and Adolescents." *Cochrane Database Systematic Reviews,* no. 7: CD008013. doi: 10.1002/14651858.CD008013.pub2.

Levin, M. 2012. "Herbal Treatment of Headache." *Headache* 52 (supp. 2): 76–80. doi: 10.1111/j.1526–4610.2012.02234.x.

Moore, R. A., et al. 2012. "Amitriptyline for Neuropathic Pain and Fibromyalgia in Adults." *Cochrane Database of Systematic Reviews,* no. 12: CD008242. doi: 10.1002/14651858.CD008242.pub2.

Orr, S. L., and S. Venkateswaran. 2014. "Nutraceuticals in the Prophylaxis of Pediatric Migraine: Evidence-Based Review and Recommendations." *Cephalalgia* 34 (8): 568–583. doi: 10.1177/0333102413519512.

Chapter 9. Additional Interventions

Adams, D., et al. 2011. "The Safety of Pediatric Acupuncture: A Systematic Review." *Pediatrics* 128 (6): e1575–e1587.

Brands, M. M., H. Purperhart, and J. M. Deckers-Kocken. 2011. "A Pilot Study of Yoga Treatment in Children with Functional Abdominal Pain and Irritable Bowel Syndrome." *Complementary Therapies in Medicine* 19 (3): 109–114.

Evans, S., et al. 2013. "Iyengar Yoga and the Use of Props for Pediatric Chronic Pain: A Case Study." *Alternative Therapies in Health and Medicine* 19 (5): 66–70.

Kundu, A., et al. 2014. "Reiki Therapy for Postoperative Oral Pain in Pediatric Patients: Pilot Data from a Double-Blind, Randomized Clinical Trial." *Complementary Therapies in Clinical Practice* 20 (1): 21–25.

Lim, A., N. Cranswick, and M. South. 2011. "Adverse Events Associated with the Use of Complementary and Alternative Medicine in Children." *Archives of Disease in Childhood* 96 (3): 297–300.

Lundeberg, T., I. Lund, and J. Näslund. 2007. "Acupuncture—Self-Appraisal and the Reward System." *Acupuncture in Medicine* 25 (3): 87–99.

Ndao, D. H., et al. 2012. "Inhalation Aromatherapy in Children and Adolescents Undergoing Stem Cell Infusion: Results of a Placebo-Controlled Double-Blind Trial." *Psychooncology* 21 (3): 247–254.

Nord, D., and J. Belew. 2009. "Effectiveness of the Essential Oils Lavender and Ginger in Promoting Children's Comfort in a Perianesthesia Setting." *Journal of Perianesthesia Nursing* 24 (5): 307–312.

O'Flaherty, L. A., et al. 2012. "Aromatherapy Massage Seems to Enhance Relaxation in Children with Burns: An Observational Pilot Study." *Burns* 38 (6): 840–845.

Smith, K. 2012. "Against Homeopathy—A Utilitarian Perspective." *Bioethics* 26 (8): 398–409.

Snyder, J., and P. Brown. 2012. "Complementary and Alternative Medicine in Children: An Analysis of the Recent Literature." *Current Opinion in Pediatrics* 24 (4): 539–546.

Vitale, A. 2007. "An Integrative Review of Reiki Touch Therapy Research." *Holistic Nursing Practice* 21 (4): 167–179; quiz 180–181.

Vohra, S., et al. 2007. "Adverse Events Associated with Pediatric Spinal Manipulation: A Systematic Review." *Pediatrics* 119 (1): e275–e283.

Zeltzer, L. 2013. "Complementary Therapy in Paediatric Pain." In *Oxford Handbook of Paediatric Pain,* edited by P. A. McGrath et al. Oxford, Eng.: Oxford University Press.

Chapter 10. A Better Breath

Bell, Katrina M., and Elizabeth A. Meadows. 2013. "Efficacy of a Brief Relaxation Training Intervention for Pediatric Recurrent Abdominal Pain." *Cognitive and Behavioral Practice* 20 (1): 81–92.

Busch, V., et al. 2012. "The Effect of Deep and Slow Breathing on Pain Perception, Autonomic Activity, and Mood Processing—An Experimental Study." *Pain Medicine* 13 (2): 215–228.

Chalaye, P., et al. 2009. "Respiratory Effects on Experimental Heat Pain and Cardiac Activity." *Pain Medicine* 10 (8): 1334–1340.

Connell, A. M., et al. 2011. "Maternal Depression and the Heart of Parenting: Respiratory Sinus Arrhythmia and Affective Dynamics during Parent-Adolescent Interactions." *Journal of Family Psychology* 25 (5): 653–662.

Dovey, Terence M., et al. 2008. "Food Neophobia and 'Picky/Fussy' Eating in Children: A Review." *Appetite* 50 (2–3): 181–193.

Harris, V. A., et al. 1976. "Paced Respiration as a Technique for the Modification of Autonomic Response to Stress." *Psychophysiology* 13 (5): 386–391.

Howard, A. J., et al. 2012. "Toddlers' Food Preferences: The Impact of Novel Food Exposure, Maternal Preferences and Food Neophobia." *Appetite* 59 (3): 818–825.

Zautra, A. J., et al. 2010. "The Effects of Slow Breathing on Affective Responses to Pain Stimuli: An Experimental Study." *Pain* 149 (1): 12–18.

Chapter 11. Connecting Mind to Body through Story

Brown, J. M. 1984. "Imagery Coping Strategies in the Treatment of Migraine." *Pain* 18 (2): 157–167.

Derbyshire, S. W., M. G. Whalley, and D. A. Oakley. 2009. "Fibromyalgia Pain and Its Modulation by Hypnotic and Non-Hypnotic Suggestion: An fMRI Analysis." *European Journal of Pain* 13 (5): 542–550.

Dobson, C. E., and M. W. Byrne. 2014. "Original Research: Using Guided Imagery to Manage Pain in Young Children with Sickle Cell Disease." *American Journal of Nursing* 114 (4): 26–36; tests 37, 47.

Kosslyn, S. M., G. Ganis, and W. L. Thompson. 2001. "Neural Foundations of Imagery." *Nature Reviews Neuroscience* 2 (9): 635–642.

Menzies, V., A. G. Taylor, and C. Bourguignon. 2006. "Effects of Guided Imagery on Outcomes of Pain, Functional Status, and Self-Efficacy in Persons Diagnosed with Fibromyalgia." *Journal of Alternative and Complementary Medicine* 12 (1): 23–30.

Moseley, G. L., and A. Arntz. 2007. "The Context of a Noxious Stimulus Affects the Pain It Evokes." *Pain* 133 (1–3): 64–71.

Posadzki, P., and E. Ernst. 2011. "Guided Imagery for Musculoskeletal Pain: A Systematic Review." *Clinical Journal of Pain* 27 (7): 648–653.

Posadzki, P., et al. 2012. "Guided Imagery for Non-Musculoskeletal Pain: A Systematic Review of Randomized Clinical Trials." *Journal of Pain Symptom Management* 44 (1): 95–104.

Rutten, J. M., et al. 2014. "Gut-Directed Hypnotherapy in Children with Irritable Bowel Syndrome or Functional Abdominal Pain (Syndrome): A Randomized Controlled Trial on Self Exercises at Home Using CD versus Individual Therapy by Qualified Therapists." *BMC Pediatrics* 14: 140.

van Tilburg, M. A., et al. 2009. "Audio-Recorded Guided Imagery Treatment Reduces Functional Abdominal Pain in Children: A Pilot Study." *Pediatrics* 124 (5): e890–e897.

Chapter 12. Targeting Muscle Tension

Conrad, A., and W. T. Roth. 2007. "Muscle Relaxation Therapy for Anxiety Disorders: It Works, But How?" *Journal of Anxiety Disorders* 21 (3): 243–264.

Finney, Jack W., et al. 1989. "Pediatric Psychology in Primary Health Care: Brief Targeted Therapy for Recurrent Abdominal Pain." *Behavior Therapy* 20 (2): 283–291.

Larsson, B., et al. 2005. "Relaxation Treatment of Adolescent Headache Sufferers: Results from a School-Based Replication Series." *Headache* 45 (6): 692–704.

Pifarré, P., et al. 2014. "Diazepam and Jacobson's Progressive Relaxation Show Similar Attenuating Short-Term Effects on Stress-Related Brain Glucose Consumption." *European Psychiatry* 30(2).

Pluess, M., A. Conrad, and F. H. Wilhelm. 2009. "Muscle Tension in Generalized Anxiety Disorder: A Critical Review of the Literature." *Journal of Anxiety Disorders* 23 (1): 1–11.

Chapter 13. One Mindful Moment at a Time

Evans, S., et al. 2008. "Mindfulness-Based Cognitive Therapy for Generalized Anxiety Disorder." *Journal of Anxiety Disorders* 22 (4): 716–721.

Grossman, P., et al. 2004. "Mindfulness-Based Stress Reduction and Health Benefits: A Meta-Analysis." *Journal of Psychosomatic Research* 57 (1): 35–43.

Lush, E., et al. 2009. "Mindfulness Meditation for Symptom Reduction in Fibromyalgia: Psychophysiological Correlates." *Journal of Clinical Psychology in Medical Settings* 16 (2): 200–207.

McCracken, L. M., J. Gauntlett-Gilbert, and K. E. Vowles. 2007. "The Role of Mindfulness in a Contextual Cognitive-Behavioral Analysis of Chronic Pain-Related Suffering and Disability." *Pain* 131 (1–2): 63–69.

McCracken, L. M., and K. E. Vowles. 2014. "Acceptance and Commitment Therapy and Mindfulness for Chronic Pain: Model, Process, and Progress." *American Psychologist* 69 (2): 178–187.

Morone, N. E., et al. 2008. "'I Felt Like a New Person': The Effects of Mindfulness Meditation on Older Adults with Chronic Pain: Qualitative Narrative Analysis of Diary Entries." *Journal of Pain* 9 (9): 841–848.

Petter, M., et al. 2014. "The Effects of Mindful Attention and State Mindfulness on Acute Experimental Pain among Adolescents." *Journal of Pediatric Psychology* 39 (5): 521–531.

Pradhan, E. K., et al. 2007. "Effect of Mindfulness-Based Stress Reduction in Rheumatoid Arthritis Patients." *Arthritis and Rheumatology* 57 (7): 1134–1142.

Rosenzweig, S., et al. 2010. "Mindfulness-Based Stress Reduction for Chronic Pain Conditions: Variation in Treatment Outcomes and Role of Home Meditation Practice." *Journal of Psychosomatic Research* 68 (1): 29–36.

Schutze, R., et al. 2010. "Low Mindfulness Predicts Pain Catastrophizing in a Fear-Avoidance Model of Chronic Pain." *Pain* 148 (1): 120–127.

Zeidan, F., et al. 2010. "The Effects of Brief Mindfulness Meditation Training on Experimentally Induced Pain." *Journal of Pain* 11 (3): 199–209.

Zeidan, F., Martucci, K. T., et al. 2011. "Brain Mechanisms Supporting the Modulation of Pain by Mindfulness Meditation." *Journal of Neuroscience* 31 (14): 5540–5548.

Chapter 14. Biofeedback

Blume, H. K., L. N. Brockman, and C. C. Breuner. 2012. "Biofeedback Therapy for Pediatric Headache: Factors Associated with Response." *Headache* 52 (9): 1377–1386.

Myrvik, M. P., A. D. Campbell, and J. L. Butcher. 2012. "Single-Session Biofeedback-Assisted Relaxation Training in Children with Sickle Cell Disease." *Journal of Pediatric Hematology-Oncology* 34 (5): 340–343.

Nestoriuc, Y., et al. 2008. "Biofeedback Treatment for Headache Disorders: A Comprehensive Efficacy Review." *Applied Psychophysiology and Biofeedback* 33 (3): 125–140.

Palermo, T. M., et al. 2009. "Randomized Controlled Trial of an Internet-Delivered Family Cognitive-Behavioral Therapy Intervention for Children and Adolescents with Chronic Pain." *Pain* 146 (1–2): 205–213.

Powers, S. W., et al. 2001. "A Pilot Study of One-Session Biofeedback Training in Pediatric Headache." *Neurology* 56 (1): 133.

Schurman, J. V., et al. 2010. "A Pilot Study to Assess the Efficacy of Biofeedback-Assisted Relaxation Training as an Adjunct Treatment for Pediatric Functional Dyspepsia Associated with Duodenal Eosinophilia." *Journal of Pediatric Psychology* 35 (8): 837–847.

Shiri, S., et al. 2013. "A Virtual Reality System Combined with Biofeedback for Treating Pediatric Chronic Headache—A Pilot Study." *Pain Medicine* 14 (5): 621–627.

Chapter 15. Supporting Your Child with Scaffolding

Baer, J. S., and P. L. Peterson. 2002. "Motivational Interviewing with Adolescents and Young Adults." In *Motivational Interviewing: Preparing People for Change,* edited by W. R. Miller and S. Rollnick. New York: Guilford Press.

Claar, R. L., L. S. Walker, and C. A. Smith. 1999. "Functional Disability in Adolescents and Young Adults with Symptoms of Irritable Bowel Syndrome: The Role of Academic, Social, and Athletic Competence." *Journal of Pediatric Psychology* 24 (3): 271–280.

Cushing, Christopher C., et al. 2014. "Meta-Analysis of Motivational Interviewing for Adolescent Health Behavior: Efficacy beyond Substance Use." *Journal of Consulting and Clinical Psychology* 82 (6): 1212.

Kravtsova, E. E. 2009. "The Cultural-Historical Foundations of the Zone of Proximal Development." *Journal of Russian and East European Psychology* 47 (6): 9–24.

Simons, Laura E., and Karen J. Kaczynski. 2012. "The Fear Avoidance Model of Chronic Pain: Examination for Pediatric Application." *Journal of Pain* 13 (9): 827–835.

Chapter 16. A Balanced Approach to the Problem of School

Boutilier, J., and S. King. 2013. "Missed Opportunities: School as an Undervalued Site for Effective Pain Management." *Pediatric Pain Letter* 15 (1): 9–16.

Claar, R. L., L. S. Walker, and C. A. Smith. 1999. "Functional Disability in Adolescents and Young Adults with Symptoms of Irritable Bowel Syndrome: The Role of Academic, Social, and Athletic Competence." *Journal of Pediatric Psychology* 24 (3): 271–280.

Dick, B. D., and R. Pillai Riddell. 2010. "Cognitive and School Functioning in Children and Adolescents with Chronic Pain: A Critical Review." *Pain Research and Management* 15 (4): 238–244.

Haraldstad, K., et al. 2011. "Pain in Children and Adolescents: Prevalence, Impact on Daily Life, and Parents' Perception—A School Survey." *Scandinavian Journal of Caring Sciences* 25 (1): 27–36.

Kearney, Christopher A. 2001. *School Refusal Behavior in Youth: A Functional Approach to Assessment and Treatment.* Washington, D.C.: American Psychological Association.

———. 2007. *Getting Your Child to Say "Yes" to School.* Oxford, Eng.: Oxford University Press.

———. 2008. "School Absenteeism and School Refusal Behavior in Youth: A Contemporary Review." *Clinical Psychology Review* 28 (3): 451–471.

Konijnenberg, A. Y., et al. 2005. "Children with Unexplained Chronic Pain: Substantial Impairment in Everyday Life." *Archives of Disease in Childhood* 90: 680–686.

Logan, D. E., R. M. Coakley, and L. Scharff. 2007. "Teachers' Perceptions of and Responses to Adolescents with Chronic Pain Syndromes." *Journal of Pediatric Psychology* 32 (2): 139–149.

Logan, D. E., et al. 2008. "School Impairment in Adolescents with Chronic Pain." *Journal of Pain* 9 (5): 407–416.

Logan, Deirdre E., Laura E. Simons, and Elizabeth A. Carpino. 2012. "Too Sick for School? Parent Influences on School Functioning among Children with Chronic Pain." *Pain* 153 (2): 437–443.

Vervoort, T., et al. 2014. "Severity of Pediatric Pain in Relation to School-Related Functioning and Teacher Support: An Epidemiological Study among School-Aged Children and Adolescents." *Pain* 155 (6): 1118–1127.

Chapter 17. Reversing the Habits of Poor Sleep

Bromberg, M. H., K. M. Gil, and L. E. Schanberg. 2012. "Daily Sleep Quality and Mood as Predictors of Pain in Children with Juvenile Polyarticular Arthritis." *Health Psychology* 31 (2): 202–209.

Dewald-Kaufmann, J. F., F. J. Oort, and A. M. Meijer. 2014. "The Effects of Sleep Extension and Sleep Hygiene Advice on Sleep and Depressive Symptoms in Adolescents: A Randomized Controlled Trial." *Journal of Child Psychology and Psychiatry* 55 (3): 273–283.

Fitzgerald, C. T., E. Messias, and D. J. Buysse. 2011. "Teen Sleep and Suicidality: Results from the Youth Risk Behavior Surveys of 2007 and 2009." *Journal of Clinical Sleep Medicine* 7 (4): 351–356.

Garaulet, M., et al. 2011. "Short Sleep Duration Is Associated with Increased Obesity Markers in European Adolescents: Effect of Physical Activity and Dietary Habits." The HELENA Study. *International Journal of Obesity (London)* 35 (10): 1308–1317.

Gibson, E. S., et al. 2006. "'Sleepiness' Is Serious in Adolescence: Two Surveys of 3,235 Canadian Students." *BMC Public Health* 6: 116.

Gilman, D. K., et al. 2007. "Primary Headache and Sleep Disturbances in Adolescents." *Headache* 47 (8): 1189–1194.

Irwin, M. R., et al. 2006. "Sleep Deprivation and Activation of Morning Levels of Cellular and Genomic Markers of Inflammation." *Archives of Internal Medicine* 166 (16): 1756–1762.

Jungquist, C. R., et al. 2010. "The Efficacy of Cognitive-Behavioral Therapy for Insomnia in Patients with Chronic Pain." *Sleep Medicine* 11 (3): 302–309.

Kim, C. W., et al. 2012. "Weekend Catch-up Sleep Is Associated with Decreased Risk of Being Overweight among Fifth-Grade Students with Short Sleep Duration." *Journal of Sleep Research* 21 (5): 546–551.

Leger, D., et al. 2012. "Total Sleep Time Severely Drops during Adolescence." *PLoS One* 7 (10): e45204.

Logan, D. E., et al. 2014. "Changes in Sleep Habits in Adolescents during Intensive Interdisciplinary Pediatric Pain Rehabilitation." *Journal of Youth and Adolescence* 44 (2): 543–555.

Manfredini, D., et al. 2013. "Prevalence of Sleep Bruxism in Children: A Systematic Review of the Literature." *Journal of Oral Rehabilitation* 40 (8): 631–642.

Marcus, C. L., et al. 2012. "Diagnosis and Management of Childhood Obstructive Sleep Apnea Syndrome." *Pediatrics* 130 (3): e714–e755.

Mitchell, M. D., et al. 2012. "Comparative Effectiveness of Cognitive Behavioral Therapy for Insomnia: A Systematic Review." *BMC Family Practice* 13: 40.

Moore, B. A., et al. 2007. "Brief Report: Evaluating the Bedtime Pass Program for Child Resistance to Bedtime—A Randomized, Controlled Trial." *Journal of Pediatric Psychology* 32 (3): 283–287.

Moore, M. 2010. "Bedtime Problems and Night Wakings: Treatment of Behavioral Insomnia of Childhood." *Journal of Clinical Psychology* 66 (11): 1195–1204.

Mullington, J. M., et al. 2010. "Sleep Loss and Inflammation." *Best Practice and Research: Clinical Endocrinology and Metabolism* 24 (5): 775–784.

Nozoe, K. T., et al. 2014. "The Role of Sleep in Juvenile Idiopathic Arthritis Patients and Their Caregivers." *Pediatric Rheumatology Online Journal* 12: 20.

Owens, J., et al. 1999. "Television-Viewing Habits and Sleep Disturbance in School Children." *Pediatrics* 104 (3): e27.

Palermo, T. M., et al. 2007. "Objective and Subjective Assessment of Sleep in Adolescents with Chronic Pain Compared to Healthy Adolescents." *Clinical Journal of Pain* 23 (9): 812–820.

———. 2011. "Behavioral and Psychosocial Factors Associated with Insomnia in Adolescents with Chronic Pain." *Pain* 152 (1): 89–94.

Palma, B. D., et al. 2006. "Effects of Sleep Deprivation on the Development of Autoimmune Disease in an Experimental Model of Systemic Lupus Erythematosus." *American Journal of Physiology: Regulatory, Integrative, and Comparative Physiology* 291 (5): R1527–R1532.

Regestein, Q., et al. 2010. "Sleep Debt and Depression in Female College Students." *Psychiatry Research* 176 (1): 34–39.

Roberts, R. E., C. R. Roberts, and Y. Xing. 2011. "Restricted Sleep among Adolescents: Prevalence, Incidence, Persistence, and Associated Factors." *Behavioral Sleep Medicine* 9 (1): 18–30.

Taylor, D. J., and B. M. Roane. 2010. "Treatment of Insomnia in Adults and Children: A Practice-Friendly Review of Research." *Journal of Clinical Psychology* 66 (11): 1137–1147.

Valrie, Cecelia R., et al. 2013. "A Systematic Review of Sleep in Pediatric Pain Populations." *Journal of Developmental and Behavioral Pediatrics* 34 (2): 120–128.

Wells, J. C., et al. 2008. "Sleep Patterns and Television Viewing in Relation to Obesity and Blood Pressure: Evidence from an Adolescent Brazilian Birth Cohort." *International Journal of Obesity (London)* 32 (7): 1042–1049.

Chapter 18. Where Are My Child's Friends?

Bravo, L., et al. 2013. "Social Stress Exacerbates the Aversion to Painful Experiences in Rats Exposed to Chronic Pain: The Role of the Locus Coeruleus." *Pain* 154 (10): 2014–2023.

Forgeron, P. A., et al. 2010. "Social Functioning and Peer Relationships in Children and Adolescents with Chronic Pain: A Systematic Review." *Pain Research and Management* 15 (1): 27–41.

Greco, L. A., K. E. Freeman, and L. Dufton. 2007. "Overt and Relational Victimization among Children with Frequent Abdominal Pain: Links to Social Skills, Academic Functioning, and Health Service Use." *Journal of Pediatric Psychology* 32 (3): 319–329.

Kashikar-Zuck, S., et al. 2007. "Social Functioning and Peer Relationships of Adolescents with Juvenile Fibromyalgia Syndrome." *Arthritis Care and Research* 57 (3): 474–480.

Palermo, T. M. 2000. "Impact of Recurrent and Chronic Pain on Child and Family Daily Functioning: A Critical Review of the Literature." *Journal of Developmental and Behavioral Pediatrics* 21 (1): 58–69.

Perquin, C. W., et al. 2000. "Pain in Children and Adolescents: A Common Experience." *Pain* 87: 51–58.

Simons, L. E., et al. 2010. "The Relation of Social Functioning to School Impairment among Adolescents with Chronic Pain." *Clinical Journal of Pain* 26 (1): 16–22.

StopBullying.gov. 2014. U.S. Department of Health and Human Services website at http://www.stopbullying.gov (accessed August 21, 2014).

Stryve. 2014. Center for Disease Control (CDC) website at http: //veto violence.cdc.gov/stryve (accessed August 21, 2014).

Chapter 19. Family Matters

Buskila, Dan. 2007. "Genetics of Chronic Pain States." *Best Practice and Research: Clinical Rheumatology* 21 (3): 535–547.

Campo, J. V., et al. 2007. "Physical and Emotional Health of Mothers of Youth with Functional Abdominal Pain." *Archives of Pediatric and Adolescent Medicine* 161 (2): 131–137.

Cano, S., M. Gillis, and W. Heinz. 2004. "Marital Functioning, Chronic Pain, and Psychological Distress." *Pain* 107 (1–2): 167–175.

Claar, Robyn Lewis, Laura E. Simons, and Deirdre E. Logan. 2008. "Parental Response to Children's Pain: The Moderating Impact of Children's Emotional Distress on Symptoms and Disability." *Pain* 138 (1): 172–179.

Connelly, M., et al. 2010. "Parent Pain Responses as Predictors of Daily Activities and Mood in Children with Juvenile Idiopathic Arthritis: The Utility of Electronic Diaries." *Journal of Pain Symptom Management* 39 (3): 579–590.

Darlington, A. S., et al. 2012. "The Influence of Maternal Vulnerability and Parenting Stress on Chronic Pain in Adolescents in a General Population Sample: The TRAILS Study." *European Journal of Pain* 16 (1): 150–159.

Eccleston, Christopher, et al. 2004. "Adolescent Chronic Pain: Patterns and Predictors of Emotional Distress in Adolescents with Chronic Pain and Their Parents." *Pain* 108 (3): 221–229.

Gerber, W. D., et al. 2010. "MIPAS-Family-Evaluation of a New Multi-Modal Behavioral Training Program for Pediatric Headaches: Clinical Effects and the Impact on Quality of Life." *Journal of Headache Pain* 11 (3): 215–225.

Henstrom, M., et al. 2014. "NPSR1 Polymorphisms Influence Recurrent Abdominal Pain in Children: A Population-Based Study." *Neurogastroenterology and Motility,* 26 (10): 1417–1425.

Hoftun, G. B., P. R. Romundstad, and M. Rygg. 2013. "Association of Parental Chronic Pain with Chronic Pain in the Adolescent and Young Adult: Family Linkage Data from the Hunt Study." *JAMA Pediatrics* 167 (1): 61–69.

Hunfeld, J. A., et al. 2002. "Physically Unexplained Chronic Pain and Its Impact on Children and Their Families: The Mother's Perception." *Psychology and Psychotherapy* 75 (3): 251–260.

Law, E. F., et al. 2014. "Systematic Review and Meta-Analysis: Parent and Family-Based Interventions for Children and Adolescents with Chronic Medical Conditions." *Journal of Pediatric Psychology* 39 (8): 866–886.

Lewandowski, A. S., et al. 2010. "Systematic Review of Family Functioning in Families of Children and Adolescents with Chronic Pain." *Journal of Pain* 11 (11): 1027–1038.

Lier, R., T. Nilsen, and P. Mork. 2014. "Parental Chronic Pain in Relation to Chronic Pain in Their Adult Offspring: Family-Linkage within the HUNT study, Norway." *BMC Public Health* 14 (797).

Lustig, J. L., et al. 1996. "Mental Health of Mothers of Children with Juvenile Rheumatoid Arthritis: Appraisal as a Mediator." *Journal of Pediatric Psychology* 21 (5): 719–733.

Palermo, Tonya M., and Christopher Eccleston. 2009. "Parents of Children and Adolescents with Chronic Pain." *Pain* 146 (1): 15–17.

Palermo, Tonya M., Cecelia R. Valrie, and Cynthia W. Karlson. 2014. "Family and Parent Influences on Pediatric Chronic Pain: A Developmental Perspective." *American Psychologist* 69 (2): 142–152.

Ramchandani, Paul G., et al. 2006. "Early Parental and Child Predictors of Recurrent Abdominal Pain at School Age: Results of a Large Population-Based Study." *Journal of the American Academy of Child and Adolescent Psychiatry* 45 (6): 729–736.

Riggio, Heidi R., Ann Marie Valenzuela, and Dana A. Weiser. 2010. "Household Responsibilities in the Family of Origin: Relations with Self-Efficacy in Young Adulthood." *Personality and Individual Differences* 48 (5): 568–573.

Sharpe, Donald, and Lucille Rossiter. 2002. "Siblings of Children with a Chronic Illness: A Meta-Analysis." *Journal of Pediatric Psychology* 27 (8): 699–710.

Sieberg, C. B., S. Williams, and L. E. Simons. 2011. "Do Parent Protective Responses Mediate the Relation between Parent Distress and Child Functional Disability among Children with Chronic Pain?" *Journal of Pediatric Psychology* 36 (9): 1043–1051.

Walker, L. S., and J. W. Greene. 1989. "Children with Recurrent Abdominal Pain and Their Parents: More Somatic Complaints, Anxiety, and Depression Than Other Patient Families?" *Journal of Pediatric Psychology* 14: 231–234.

Index

Other Books in the Yale University Press Health & Wellness Series

Joseph A. Abboud, M.D., and Soo Kim Abboud, M.D., *No More Joint Pain*

Thomas E. Brown, Ph.D., *Attention Deficit Disorder: The Unfocused Mind in Children and Adults*

Patrick Conlon, *The Essential Hospital Handbook: How to Be an Effective Partner in a Loved One's Care*

Richard C. Frank, M.D., *Fighting Cancer with Knowledge and Hope: A Guide for Patients, Families, and Health Care Providers*

Michelle A. Gourdine, M.D., *Reclaiming Our Health: A Guide to African American Wellness*

Marjorie Greenfield, M.D., *The Working Woman's Pregnancy Book*

Ruth H. Grobstein, M.D., Ph.D., *The Breast Cancer Book: What You Need to Know to Make Informed Decisions*

James W. Hicks, M.D., *Fifty Signs of Mental Illness: A Guide to Understanding Mental Health*

Steven L. Maskin, M.D., *Reversing Dry Eye Syndrome: Practical Ways to Improve Your Comfort, Vision, and Appearance*

Mary Jane Minkin, M.D., and Carol V. Wright, Ph.D., *A Woman's Guide to Menopause and Perimenopause*

Mary Jane Minkin, M.D., and Carol V. Wright, Ph.D., *A Woman's Guide to Sexual Health*

Arthur W. Perry, M.D., F.A.C.S., *Straight Talk about Cosmetic Surgery*

Eric Pfeiffer, M.D., *Caregiving in Alzheimer's and Other Dementias*

Eric Pfeiffer, M.D., *Winning Strategies for Successful Aging*

Catherine M. Poole, with DuPont Guerry IV, M.D., *Melanoma: Prevention, Detection, and Treatment,* 2nd ed.

Madhuri Reddy, M.D., M.Sc., and Rebecca Cottrill, R.N., M.Sc.C.H. *Healing Wounds, Healthy Skin: A Practical Guide for Patients with Chronic Wounds*

E. Fuller Torrey, M.D., *Surviving Prostate Cancer: What You Need to Know to Make Informed Decisions*

Barry L. Zaret, M.D., and Genell J. Subak-Sharpe, M.S., *Heart Care for Life: Developing the Program That Works Best for You*

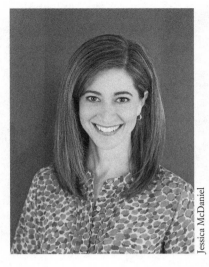

Jessica McDaniel

Rachael Coakley, Ph.D., is associate director of psychological services in the Pain Treatment Service, Department of Anesthesiology, Perioperative and Pain Medicine, Boston Children's Hospital. She is also assistant professor, Department of Psychiatry, Harvard Medical School.

Dr. Coakley specializes in providing psychological evaluation and cognitive behavioral treatment for children and adolescents coping with pain, pain-related stress, anxiety and depression. She is founder of the Comfort Ability Workshop, a supportive and interactive one-day pain-management program that introduces parents and kids to a variety of effective pain-management skills. She directs this workshop every six weeks at Boston Children's Hospital and has implemented this program at several other children's hospitals in the United States and Canada. She has also developed a self-guided video-based pain-management intervention for children with sickle cell disease and co-founded a manualized six-week group therapy program for young adults with chronic pain.

Dr. Coakley has published numerous articles and chapters on pediatric pain management and related topics. She has presented at national and international conferences and regularly speaks to parenting groups about parent-based strategies for supporting a child with chronic pain.

She is a graduate of the University of Pennsylvania and Loyola University Chicago. She lives in Boston, MA, with her husband and her two young boys who, because they really had no choice, have truly learned to love belly breathing and guided imagery. Follow her on twitter: @CoakleyRachael.